HERBAL REMEDIES

for WOMEN

AMANDA McQUADE CRAWFORD, M.N.I.M.H.

PRIMA PUBLISHING

With thanks to my soul mate, Mark. Genius drummer, inspired writer, staunch Keeper of
The Chicago Manual of Style *when I would waver . . . you understand the beauty of*
form and rhythm. From you I also learned that the greatest healer may be true love.
May all my sisters know true love and make peace on earth.

© 1997 by Amanda McQuade Crawford

PRIMA PUBLISHING and colophon are registered trademarks of Prima Communications, Inc.

Illustrations by Helene D. Stevens

Disclaimer
Prima Publishing has designed this book to provide information in regard to the subject matter covered. It is sold with the understanding that the publisher and the author are not liable for the misconception or misuse of information provided. Every effort has been made to make this book as complete and as accurate as possible. The purpose of this book is to educate. The author and Prima Publishing shall have neither liability nor responsibility to any person or entity with respect to any loss, damage, or injury caused or alleged to be caused directly or indirectly by the information contained in this book. The information presented herein is in no way intended as a substitute for medical counseling.

Library of Congress Cataloging-in-Publication Data

Crawford, Amanda McQuade.
    Herbal remedies for women : discover nature's wonderful secrets just for women / Amanda McQuade Crawford.
        p.   cm.
    Includes bibliographical references and index.
        ISBN 0-7615-0980-1
    1. Herbs—Therapeutic use. 2. Women—Diseases—Alternative treatment. I. Title.
    RM666.H33C73 1996
    615'.321'082—dc21   97-7653
                                                                       CIP

97 98 99 00 01 02 DD 10 9 8 7 6 5 4 3 2
Printed in the United States of America

How to Order
Single copies may be ordered from Prima Publishing, P.O. Box 1260BK, Rocklin, CA 95677; telephone (916) 632-4400. Quantity discounts are also available. On your letterhead, include information concerning the intended use of the books and the number of books you wish to purchase.

Visit us online at http://www.primapublishing.com

Contents

Part Four: Healthy Reproduction

Part Five: Infections

Part Six: The Change of Life

Preface

MANY WORDS HAVE been written about healing and nature over the last twenty years—or even the last ten thousand years. All herbalists, from the Ph.D.s to the bumblebees, know which herbs do what, so why write these herbal and ecological truths again? First, because there are new findings to report. In addition, there have been mistakes made in the popular media that demand a balance of more accurate herbal information. Some of us who work with herbs need to be reminded of what we already know. And there are those to whom herbal therapy is a new field. Finally, I wrote this book because I believe that the world's most helpful teachings are the same simple truths repeated in different forms, time and again, so that all may understand. It has certainly helped *me* to write "eat whole foods" a hundred times.

The herbal suggestions that I provide in this book are designed to require relatively few herbs. A woman who is new to herbs will get the best results with a manageably small list of herbs, used in several combinations for different effects. Though I will describe over two hundred herbs here, I don't expect you to buy, remember, understand, or need all of them.

The herb combinations that I recommend in this book can also be used by a willing practitioner or licensed caregiver who is learning about the use of botanical remedies with clients. These combinations are intended to be used by someone working on her own self-healing, with or without a physician's supervision, since I provide cautions where I feel they are appropriate.

In general, I prefer not to write down herbal formulas for treating particular symptoms or diseases since we treat individuals, not labels or diagnoses. I have overcome my bias to write this book, since it seems reasonable to give identifiable guidelines and clear suggestions. If you are an herbalist, I encourage you to substitute your favorite local materia medica for the herbs I recommend in a formula, as your rapport with your remedies according to your own system of practice will best serve a real-live person, no matter the pattern of disease.

In this book, I both question scientific studies and use them to back up claims for herbal or natural therapies. This is not merely a case of convenience. I love science when it increases our understanding of how things work, but the Western biomedical model is not the only way to understand disease and health. There are also abuses of so-called "scientific" information when experiments are undertaken to "prove" things that are favorable to the funding corporation.

At the end of the day, medicinal herbs cannot be judged by a Western medical rationale alone. The future of health care depends on our willingness to assess medical drugs and natural therapies according to the truth, not scientific or folkloric dogma. The truth is determined by testing whether drugs or natural therapies improve human health. When isolated compounds are tested on lab animals or in petri dishes, scientists may draw conclusions about safety that don't hold true when compounds are prescribed for people. How does testing herbs the same way drugs are tested provide dangerous misinformation? For example, beta-carotene is traditionally eaten in fruits and vegetables while the supplement has proved to be less effective. One knows the right dose for the right person by experience or following recommendations based on clinical experience. We are fortunate to be able to test herbs in their traditional context (right plant, right dose, right person). Superstition and arrogance exist on both sides of the fence separating science from traditional knowledge and use. It is time to re-fashion that fence into a bridge.

Women's health is not a separate issue from planetary health. Many conventional prescription drugs are made in factories that pour wastes into rivers and seas. Just as a "cure" requires paying attention to each individual woman, use of natural medicine means paying attention to each biological system, from the microcosm of the cell to the whole person to the global sphere. In a way, using herbs to treat common gynecological conditions heals a whole world.

This book is divided into several parts, covering menstruation and its common difficulties, abnormal cell growth, reproduction, infections, and menopause. Each chapter starts with a definition of the condition being discussed, a brief description of the issues surrounding this condition if cofactors such as stress and environment are known, cautions and conventional medical views, holistic herbal guidelines, nutrition, and additional suggestions.

I have included some overused and endangered plants when my experience indicates that they provide the most reliable treatment for a given health imbalance. However, I do point out whether a species is endangered, especially if the new consensus among herbalists is that less-endangered herbal substitutions may be appropriate.

The information found in this book reflects my truth, my training, and my experience. It is offered as a stepping stone to each who would find her own truth. May our earth be well.

Amanda McQuade Crawford
Ojai, California

Acknowledgments

THIS WORK WAS originally commissioned by Commonwoman's Health Project, a cooperative women's clinic in Santa Rosa, California. These herbal protocols were intended to be used by trained medical personnel in various women's clinics around the United States and other countries. A genuine zeal on the part of clinicians looking for safe and effective herbal therapy resulted in the forty-page manual, *Clinic Handbook of Herbal Protocols for Common Gynecological Conditions,* written by myself and Brenda Jackson, a gifted nurse practitioner. My profound thanks go to Brenda for contributing her considerable skills in bridging health treatment modalities, as well as for initiating the project.

The demand for this information from students of herbal medicine and from clients resulted in many informal editions of this gynecology manual, previously titled *Gaiacology*. For updates and corrections, I am grateful to Pat Wiley, nurse-midwife.

Developing herbal protocols in *Gaiacology* into a guide for all women has taken some years as new insights have been incorporated into an otherwise dry booklet for health professionals. The questions of my brightest students sparked new research while the answers shared by my colleagues provided confirmation about the use of whole plants for whole people.

I am indebted to my colleague and friend, Medical Herbalist Jonathan Treasure, M.N.I.M.H., who saved me considerable embarrassment by catching my mistakes, "howlers" as well as "clangers." Any errors remaining are mine alone. Thanks are also due to my patient editor Brenda Nichols. To all my teachers including my students, peers, and the herbs too. I give my thanks.

PART ONE

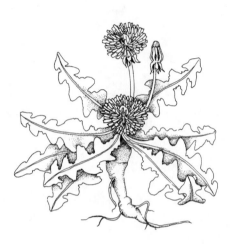

Introduction to Herbs

1

Herbal Glossary

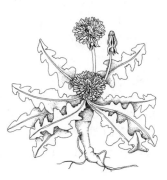

For two-thirds of the people on earth, traditional medicine is herbal medicine. Natural medicine is not an alternative; it surrounds us and it is all we have, whether we take it straight from the vine or alter it in a lab. Natural therapies are not a complement to medicine. The word *conventional* describes the Western medical approach, also called *allopathic medicine.* Allopathic medicine is not *traditional medicine,* because the latter term refers to methods far older and more global than modern Western science. Herbal medicine is one type of traditional medicine.

In the emerging model of biological sciences, the emphasis is now on *integrated medicine*—using the most appropriate method for each person, each time she needs help. In the case of a car crash or a life-threatening gynecological emergency, gentle herbal teas taken over several weeks are not the most appropriate medicine. Herbal treatment can be appropriate after the situation is stable. Good medicine means knowing what is indicated for the patient's best care. Everyone from natural therapists to surgeons can make peace with the concept of integrated or *appropriate medicine.*

What does an herb actually do in the body? From ancient times, herbalists have described the therapeutic properties of herbs in ways that explain their action to the best of our understanding. Modern terms are also used today, though the most scientific words are no more accurate than some ancient descriptive words.

Some terms describing what herbs do require a definition. The Glossary defines the words used to describe the actions of medicinal plants and explains which parts of the plant are used: roots, leaves, and so on.

Traditionally used parts of the plant are not broken down by practicing herbalists in a lab for one "active constituent" to create a drug-like standardized effect. We all know that standardized drugs from natural or synthetic sources come with a list of side effects. The complex biochemistry of a whole root, for example, may be extracted by water in a cup of tea, by alcohol and water in a *tincture,* or perhaps by oil in an herbal *salve*. Different herbs with their many active constituents are known to extract best in particular preparations. Most preparations of whole herbs are easily made at home. They are described in Chapter 2: Herbal Preparation.

In herbology, the word *action* is used to describe an herb's effects. In the section of this chapter called "Herbal Actions," I will define various herbal actions and provide a short list of herbs for each action, starting with milder herbs and ending with stronger ones. In herbal medicine it is often true that the milder the herb, the deeper the cure. The herbs I will describe here are safe herbs that I have used for years with women of all ages. When I introduce an herb that is potentially harmful, I will provide appropriate cautions. This information may not always reflect what bureaucrats, medical "experts," or threatened pharmaceutical corporations regard as safe.

Herbs that have more than one medicinal benefit appear in more than one action category. Most whole herbs (roots, leaves, seeds, flowers) have several actions, some more obvious than others. Using the appropriate part of a whole plant involves more than one chemical, having more than one effect in the body. Often, what conventional science considers to be a "less active" herb chemical turns out to be an important cofactor (a necessary compound) for that herb's therapeutic effect and safer metabolism.

Parts of Plants

Roots and *rhizomes* are underground plant parts, collected when the flowering plant is dormant in autumn or early spring. Dandelion, for example, is often used in root form. Sometimes herbalists use the outer part of the root as in the case of the rhizome *Oplopanax* (devil's club root).

Bark refers to the outer part of the above-ground plant, for example, tree bark from *Salix spp.* (willow bark). (Note: "spp." is an abbreviation of the word "species.")

Most medicinal *flowers,* such as *Calendula* (common name: calendula or pot marigold), are collected in each plant's flowering season. This is usually between late spring and late summer, after the buds open and before they blossom fully.

The general term *herb* refers to all of the above-ground parts, including the stem, leaf, and any flowers. Examples include *Mentha spp.* (mint) and *Urtica spp.* (nettle). The word "herb" can also refer to small or delicate plants, such as *Stellaria media* (chickweed) or *Galium aparine* (cleavers). The herbalist's use of the term "herb" is not the same as the botanist's because "medicinal herbs" include shrubs, even trees.

Essential oils are the same as *volatile oils*: the fragrance of a plant that evaporates with heat. These aromatic oils are extracted from herbs by steam distillation or other methods not easily managed in the home kitchen. Pure essential oils can be purchased in small amounts. They are quite pharmacologically active. Dosages for external use are counted in drops and diluted in other liquids such as bath water, aloe gel, or massage oils.

Application of aromatic plant oils can be therapeutic. *Aromatherapy* utilizes the chemical pathways of smell through the brain's emotional center, the *limbic region* and *hypothalamus* of the central nervous system. Indeed, a lavender bath is relaxing to the mind as well as the body. In aromatherapy, essential oils are only taken internally under the supervision of a qualified herbalist or aromatherapist.

The *resin* of a plant—dried drops of its sap—can also be used in herbal medicine. The resin of the myrrh tree is a good example.

Some other plant parts can be used, and I will explain those in relation to particular herbs later in the book.

Herbal Actions

These herb examples of each action are listed in order of mildest to strongest. Some herbs work in such mild ways that they are not actually defined these ways in other sources. Yet they give women the gentlest choice.

Adaptogens help us adapt to stress by supporting the adrenal glands, the endocrine system, and the whole person.

> nettle leaf (*Urtica dioica*)
>
> sarsaparilla (*Smilax ornata*)
>
> licorice root (*Glycyrrhiza glabra*)
>
> devil's club (*Oplopanax horridum*)
>
> suma root, also called "para todo" (*Pfaffia paniculata*)
>
> Siberian ginseng root (*Eleutherococcus senticosus*)
>
> ashwagandha (*Withania somnifera*)
>
> ginseng root (*Panax ginseng*)

Alteratives alter a long-standing condition by aiding the elimination of metabolic toxins. Called "blood cleansers" in the past, these herbs improve lymphatic circulation, boost immunity, and help clear chronic conditions of the skin.

> calendula flower (*Calendula officinalis*)
>
> fresh cleavers herb (*Galium aparine*)
>
> nettle leaf (*Urtica dioica*)
>
> red clover flower (*Trifolium pratense*)
>
> burdock root (*Arctium lappa*)

Analgesics or *anodynes* relieve the pain symptom. Some herbs are strong pain relievers, often working best against pains of specific causes.

lavender flower (*Lavandula vera, L. spica, and other species*): headaches

feverfew herb (*Chrysanthemum parthenium*): migraines

cabbage leaves (*Brassica spp.*): externally for mastitis

wintergreen leaf or essential oil (*Gaultheria procumbens*): externally on sore muscles

passionflower herb and flower (*Passiflora incarnata*): physical and emotional pain

cramp bark (*Viburnum opulus*): muscle pain

valerian root (*Valeriana officinalis*): muscular and nervous system pain

St. Johnswort flower, herb, and oil (*Hypericum perforatum*): flowering tops are used internally; the oil is not an essential oil but a liquid made with herb and vegetable oil, used externally on wounds and over nerves damaged in trauma

poppy flower (*Papaver somniferum*): a sedative for short-term use in severe pain

Antacids reduce excess stomach acid, helping the stomach lining recuperate to accommodate the healthy gastric acid needed for good digestion.

marshmallow root and leaf (*Althaea officinalis*): this demulcent absorbs excess acid

meadowsweet herb (*Filipendula ulmaria,* also called *Spirea ulmaria*)

hops flower (*Humulus lupulus*) (also a *bitter*; see definition following)

sweet flag (*Acorus calamus*): in low doses; ¼ teaspoon root powder or equivalent

Anticatarrhals clear excess mucus, usually working in the upper respiratory tract to help relieve congested sinus cavities, ears, nose, and throat. This special group of astringent herbs also clears discharge from other mucous-membrane-lined organs.

goldenrod herb (*Solidago virgaurea*)

lemon balm herb (*Melissa officinalis*)

yarrow flower (*Achillea millefolium*)

Antidepressants lift the mood and soothe the heart and spirit; some also stabilize emotional shifts.

lemon balm herb (*Melissa officinalis*)

lavender flower (*Lavandula vera, L. spica,* and other species)

kava kava (*Piper methysticum*)

vervain herb (*Verbena officinalis*)

St. Johnswort flower (*Hypericum perforatum*)

kola nut (*Cola vera*): contains caffeine; also a central digestive system stimulant to metabolism

Anti-emetics reduce nausea or stop vomiting.

lemon balm herb (*Melissa officinalis*): safe for use during pregnancy (usually used as a tea or syrup to avoid using alcohol tinctures during the first trimester)

black horehound herb (*Ballota nigra*): safe for use during pregnancy; stronger effect and smell than lemon balm, but tastes acceptable

ginger root (*Zingiber officinale*): safe for use during pregnancy; proven clinically to relieve motion sickness

Anti-inflammatories reduce inflammation without completely suppressing symptoms, assisting the body in self-repair from the cause of the inflammation.

chamomile flowers and essential oil (*Matricaria recutita*): accelerates wound healing; mentally calming

meadowsweet herb (*Filipendula ulmaria* also called *Spirea ulmaria*): aids digestive lining in ulceration, joint lining in arthritis

calendula flowers (*Calendula officinalis*): wound repair with antiviral protection

wild yam root (*Dioscorea villosa*): digestive anti-inflammatory, used with spasm

licorice root (*Glycyrrhiza glabra*): plant steroid activity is anti-inflammatory on contact, indirectly throughout tissues; excessive use aggravates water retention, other side effects (high blood pressure, low potassium)

Antimicrobials clear infections by strengthening natural defenses. Like antiseptics (see following description), these plants may kill off certain microorganisms directly. Some work only in certain parts of the body.

uva-ursi leaf, also called bearberry (*Arctostaphylos uva-ursi*): usually used as tea to prevent or treat urinary tract infections

yarrow herb and flower (*Achillea millefolium*): multipurpose herb helps five systems: skin, urinary, digestive, reproductive, and circulatory systems garlic clove (*Allium sativum*): broad-spectrum antimicrobial; antifungal and bactericidal; antiviral used for widespread immune-system benefits including skin, digestive, upper respiratory, and circulatory systems; lowers cholesterol levels in the blood

barberry root (*Berberis spp.*): antimicrobial, anticatarrhal, hepatic

echinacea root, seed, and flower (*Echinacea purpurea, E. angustifolia, E. pallida, E. tennesiensis*): overused by average health consumer but still valuable as a short-term immune boost

goldenseal (*Hydrastis canadensis*): broad-spectrum agent for inflamed mucous membranes

Antiseptics kill microorganisms directly and slow or stop tissue decay.

chamomile flower and herb (*Matricaria recutita*): digestion, externally on delicate skin; also calming

thyme herb (*Thymus vulgaris*): used for wet lungs, externally on bad wounds

myrrh resin (*Commiphora mol-mol*): often used as tincture on skin, digestive, upper respiratory systems against common contagious infections

Externally only:

ti tree essential oil (*Melaleuca alternifolia*): especially against fungi; sometimes spelled "tea tree," though unrelated to the tea one drinks

lavender essential oil (*Lavandula vera*): safe and effective for most skin problems, whether dry or weepy

Antispasmodics slow or stop cramps and muscle spasms.

wild yam root (*Dioscorea villosa*): for most digestive and some reproductive cramps

black haw bark (*Viburnum prunifolium*): best as tea, though also used as tincture for uterine and ovarian cramps

cramp bark (*Viburnum opulus*): strongly relaxing to all voluntary and involuntary muscles

valerian root (*Valeriana officinalis*): muscle relaxant and mental sedative

Aperients are mild laxatives, stimulating colon cleansing. These herbs relieve occasional constipation and pelvic congestion.

dandelion root (*Taraxacum officinale*)

psyllium seeds (*Plantago psyllium, P. ovata*): a bulk laxative, the seeds or seed hulls are taken with water to swell up and provide bulk to safely stimulate elimination flax seeds (*Linum usitatissimum*)

yellow dock root (*Rumex crispus*)

prunes, soaked dried fruit (*Prunus spp.*)

Astringents slow the loss of body fluids. Unlike cosmetic astringents, these herbs are taken internally and topically to tone and tighten tissues, especially membranes that are inflamed. A type of astringent called a *hemostatic* stops bleeding; an external hemostatic is called a *styptic*. Each of these astringent herbs helps with a different problem, such as diarrhea, heavy menstrual bleeding, or discharge.

yarrow flower (*Achillea millefolium*): affects several body systems; internally as tea also preventive or treatment for bloody nose; externally on skin for bleeding

horsetail herb (*Equisetum arvense*): urinary system

rose petals (*Rosa spp.*): any body system, especially digestive and reproductive

witch hazel bark (*Hamamelis virginiana*): any body system, externally on skin

partridgeberry herb, formerly squaw vine (*Mitchella repens*): reproductive, especially with pelvic congestion, as with fibroids

fresh shepherd's purse herb (*Capsella bursa-pastoris*): reproductive, especially during labor, bleeding between cycles, or flooding of menopause

oak bark (*Quercus robur*): any body system; the highest level of tannins make oak one of the strongest general astringents

Bitters improve digestive health, may relieve gas, increase appetite for healthy foods, and reduce an unhealthy appetite for sweets. These are often *hepatics* (see following description). The bitter flavor changes sluggishness to activity, improving elimination, and assisting antidepressants in lifting the body and mind.

chamomile flower (*Matricaria recutita*)

chicory root (*Cichorium intybus*)

dandelion root and leaf (*Taraxacum officinale*)

calendula flower (*Calendula officinalis*)

yarrow flower (*Achillea millefolium*)

motherwort herb (*Leonurus cardiaca*)

yellow dock root (*Rumex crispus*)

vervain herb (*Verbena officinalis*)

mugwort herb (*Artemisia vulgaris*)

Cardiovascular tonics strengthen the heart and blood vessels. Some regulate blood vessel tone and strengthen cardiac muscle, while others give a person "heart" and courage for better endurance.

borage flower (*Borago officinalis*): traditionally given as the "gladdening herb" for sadness or to increase joy

linden tree leaf and flowers, also called lime tree, though not related to citrus (*Tilia platyphylla, T. europea*): given especially when there is also digestive inflammation

motherwort herb (*Leonurus cardiaca*): best for rapid heart beat and anxiety

hawthorn flowers, leaf, and berry (*Crataegus monogyna, C. oxyacantha*)

ginkgo leaf (*Ginkgo biloba*): used for cardiovascular and nervous system tone

garlic clove (*Allium sativum*): for high cholesterol and immune-system benefits

Carminatives clear up gas and bloating by sweetening the intestines with aromatic oils. They are mild antiseptics (they slow or stop decay by normalizing intestinal flora) and antispasmodics (they reduce spasms by bringing circulating blood to warm and soothe the intestines).

lemon balm (*Melissa officinalis*)

chamomile flower (*Matricaria recutita*)

peppermint leaf (*Mentha piperita*)

cardamom seed (*Elettaria cardamomum*)

fennel seed (*Foeniculum vulgare*)

aniseed, anise seed (*Pimpinella anisum*)

dill seed (*Anethum graveolens*)

caraway seed (*Carum carvi*)

ginger root (*Zingiber officinale*)

Demulcents soothe inflamed surfaces, inside or out, and provide nourishment.

corn silk (*Zea mays*): the thin yellow hairs between the corn and the tough outer green husk contain plant sugars that soothe the urinary tract

plantain leaf and seed (*Plantago major, P. minor, P. ovata*): for adding movement and moisture to any body system, especially respiratory and digestive, and externally on skin

marshmallow root (*Althaea officinalis*): for entire digestive tract, dry coughs
in the lungs, and irritated urinary tract

slippery elm bark (*Ulmus fulva*): used especially for mouth, throat, and
stomach and colon irritation

aloe gel, pulp inside leaf (*Aloe vera*): used externally for burns, internally
for raw digestive tract

comfrey root and leaf (*Symphytum officinale*): used externally for any skin or
vaginal irritation; internally for six or eight weeks at a time for adults
to speed healing of broken bones

Diaphoretics increase perspiration by helping the sweat glands open and increasing peripheral blood flow so that the body may sweat out impurities and cool
down to a normal temperature. They are usually best given as a hot tea.

yarrow flower (*Achillea millefolium*)

elder flower (*Sambucus nigra*)

boneset herb (*Eupatorium perfoliatum*): bitter tonic especially for the flu or
"twenty-four-hour bugs" with any digestive symptoms

Diuretics increase the volume of urine passed to help correct bloating and
water retention.

corn silk (*Zea mays*)

marshmallow leaf and root (*Althaea officinalis*)

yarrow flower (*Achillea millefolium*)

parsley leaf (*Petroselinum crispum*)

horsetail herb (*Equisetum arvense*)

uva-ursi leaf, also called bearberry (*Arctostaphylos uva-ursi*)

Emmenagogues is a term some use to mean any herb stimulating reproductive
function. In this book, the term is limited to herbs that cause endometrial shedding;
they stimulate normal menstrual cycles in the absence of pregnancy (please see
"Herbs to Avoid During Pregnancy" in Chapter 15).

partridgeberry herb, formerly squaw vine (*Mitchella repens*)

yarrow flower (*Achillea millefolium*)

vitex, also called chaste tree or chasteberry seed (*Vitex agnus-castus*)

pennyroyal (*Mentha pulegium*): this minty herb tea is safe and helpful for
young girls with delayed menses due to travel or sickness; the essential
oil available in some stores is not safe internally at all, ever

mugwort herb (*Artemisia vulgaris*): a bitter herb that stimulates normal appetite and flow of blocked menstrual material due to tension, and is mildly relaxing

Galactagogues increase the quantity of breast milk during lactation.

anise seed, also aniseed (*Pimpinella anisum*): as tea, also given to mother for colicky baby

fennel herb and seed (*Foeniculum vulgare*)

milk thistle seed (*Carduus marianum*, also *Silybum marianum*): used when difficulty with breast-feeding is combined with liver damage

vervain herb (*Verbena officinalis*): a strong bitter that helps the flow of milk by stimulating liver and digestion, though it is emotionally relaxing; safe during breast-feeding, it is not recommended during pregnancy

Hepatics promote liver health and gallbladder function by improving fat metabolism via the production of bile (*cholagogue*) and increased flow of bile (*choleretic*); other liver functions improved by hepatic herbs

dandelion root and leaf (*Taraxacum officinale*)

motherwort herb (*Leonurus cardiaca*)

hops flower (*Humulus lupulus*)

milk thistle (*Carduus marianum* also *Silybum marianum*): protects and repairs liver cells

fringe tree bark (*Chionanthus virginicus*): especially given when gallstones and jaundice are present

goldenseal root (*Hydrastis canadensis*): a strong plant reserved for the liver with immune damage

Hypnotics send us to sleep but do not cause a hypnotic trance; the name comes from the Greek god of sweet dreams, Hypnos.

chamomile (*Matricaria recutita*)

passionflower herb (*Passiflora incarnata*)

wild lettuce leaf (*Lactuca virosa*)

hops flower (*Humulus lupulus*)

valerian root (*Valeriana officinalis*)

Hormonal tonics normalize or balance levels of estrogen and other hormones by affecting the feedback regulation of the endocrine system, assisting natural functioning, and reversing infertility, irregular menstrual cycles, and the effects of the birth-control pill.

sarsaparilla root (*Smilax ornata*): helps with lymph and chronic reproductive imbalances

red clover flower (*Trifolium pratense*): calming and mineralizing herb with some protective phytosterols

black cohosh root (*Cimicifuga racemosa*): antispasmodic with estrogenic effects, given with nervous system pain or tension

vitex, also called chaste tree or chasteberry seed (*Vitex agnus-castus*): raises luteinizing hormone levels by maintaining the corpus luteum after ovulation

dong quai, also tang kwei root (*Angelica sinensis*): raises estrogenic effects; may paradoxically lower excess estrogen through complex feedback mechanisms

saw palmetto berry (*Serenoa serrulata or S. repens*): slows the enzymatic change of testosterone to its stronger version, 5-alpha dihydrotestoterone) in both women and men

Nervines affect the nerves. They are a large group of herbs that include relaxants, nutritive tonics, and even stimulants, such as the well-known coffee bean (*Coffea arabica, C. spp.*), with both its good and ill effects.

Nervine relaxants safely reduce anxiety and tension, also relieving irritability and the effects of stress on the body.

linden flower (*Tilia europea*)

chamomile flower (*Matricaria recutita*)

hyssop herb (*Hyssopus officinalis*)

lavender flower (*Lavandula vera, L. spica, and other species*)

motherwort herb (*Leonurus cardiaca*)

skullcap herb (*Scutellaria lateriflora*)

passionflower (*Passiflora incarnata*)

hops flower (*Humulus lupulus*)

Nervine stimulants stimulate nerves, giving quick energy.

peppermint (*Mentha piperita*)

kola (*Cola vera*): contains stimulating alkaloid caffeine

Nervine tonics nourish nerve tissue and can be taken whether or not one has a "nerve problem."

oat straw and seed (*Avena sativa*)

skullcap herb (*Scutellaria lateriflora*)

vervain herb (*Verbena officinalis*)

damiana leaf (*Turnera diffusa*)

ginkgo leaf (*Ginkgo biloba*)

St. Johnswort flower (*Hypericum perforatum*)

Uterine tonics benefit reproductive health, especially after surgery, giving birth, or chronic ill health. Some uterine tonics act hormonally, some do not.

raspberry leaf (*Rubus idaeus*): reproduction

partridgeberry herb, formerly called squaw vine (*Mitchella repens*)

blue cohosh root (*Caulophyllum thalictroides*): astringent and antispasmodic given for self-repair with tissue overgrowth or damage

Vulneraries heal wounds or inflammation inside or out, often by disinfecting while knitting cells together, resulting in less scarring.

plantain leaf (*Plantago major, P. minor, P. ovata*)

chamomile flower (*Matricaria recutita*)

calendula flower (*Calendula officinalis*)

yarrow flower (*Achillea millefolium*)

St. Johnswort herb (*Hypericum perforatum*)

comfrey leaf (*Symphytum officinale*)

myrrh resin (*Commiphora mol-mol*)

Remember: while an herb may be considered mild *in comparison* to the others listed after it, it may have profound healing effects.

There is a mistaken notion these days that herbs are weak and so large quantities are needed. Even mild herbs have more than one action, so as a guideline, use the combinations for specific conditions found in this book. Because these are safe for home experimentation within recommended limits, you may choose your own medicine, but beware the pitfall of taking too many "beneficial" things. Start your healing journey with one, two, or at the most three plants, according to your needs and each herb's "bouquet" of actions. When in doubt, leave it out—or better yet, ask an herbalist.

2
Herbal Preparation

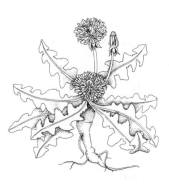

How does one take herbs? Should one make herb tea, take a tincture, or buy capsules? Beginning herb students are often dismayed at an experienced herbalist's answer: "It depends." There is both a science and an art to preparing herbs. You may take herbs in food (garlic, basil), as tea (chamomile, rose hips), in capsules (pau d'arco), as liquid tinctures, as liquid extracts (even more concentrated than tinctures), or as external massage liniments and oils. You can even absorb herbs through your skin in a hot bath.

In this chapter, I will describe common forms of herbal preparation.

Harvesting

First, only collect an herb in the wild if you are certain that you recognize it as the correct species. Many wonderful herbs have nonmedicinal or even potentially toxic look-alikes that may confuse someone new to field identification. Plants outdoors look different from pictures in a book. Their identifying signs (number of leaflets, arrangement of flower parts) can be learned, but superficial appearances vary naturally due to soil composition, time of year, rainfall, and other factors.

To get closer to your medicine, buy a handbook for field identification (see Bibliography) or go on herb walks with a botanist, herbalist, or other person experienced with identification. Contact your nearest wildflower society through your local telephone book to find the experts nearest home.

Second, as a result of ecological damage caused by enthusiastic herb pickers, some valuable herbs have been reclassified as threatened or endangered. The ones that get all the media attention are threatened first. Though some herbs are precious, we are not dependent on the latest darling of the popular media. We are meant to know a handful of alternatives so that our needs can be met without depleting the plant communities.

Professional herb growers have developed standards for environmentally conscious harvesting. Buying herbs from them rewards both ethical herb growers and the earth itself. For further information, see "Resources."

Collecting

You should collect leaves, flowers, or flowering tops using clippers, pruning shears, or scissors—not by breaking off or tearing, which allows disease to invade the remaining plant. Collect herbs during dry weather, after the dew of the morning has evaporated, and before the midday full sun.

When collecting leaves, cut off whole stems just below a leaf to allow new growth. Later, you can strip off dry leaves. In one collection visit, take no more than enough to loosely fill one paper grocery bag.

Different flowers are best collected at different stages for maximum medicinal effect, especially when volatile oil content is a factor. Collect flowers such as chamomile or yarrow just before they are fully open, for example. Take no more at one time than will fill your kitchen colander; leave some for the bees, butterflies, and other insects.

Fruits are collected in autumn when they are fully grown, but not always fully ripe, so that their fruit acids and other constituents are preserved before the ripe pulp withers on the vine. Examples of such fruits are hawthorn berries and rose hips. Remember to leave some for the birds and small animals.

Seeds are collected in dry weather when mature. They are usually ready to drop, all dry, from fruits that have split open in late summer. Examples are anise and fennel, taken when mature for mellow volatile oils. Leave some to allow new plants to grow.

Barks are collected when the tree or shrub is inactive: early spring before sap rises or autumn when the plant is going dormant. Always take off patches in small vertical strips; never take off a ring that encircles the tree, or it will die.

Roots and underground bulbs are collected when the plant has not begun to flower, since by then all the energy has left the root and gone into reproductive flower parts. An example is the annual garlic. Perennials are collected after a minimum of two to three years of growth (longer for the ginseng family and many others), in the spring or fall. Tap roots such as dandelion are not collected at the height of growth (summer) because they will shrink and stay spongy on drying.

Collect the plant parts that seem ready to be collected. Outer criteria for readiness include an absence of bug bites, moldy spots, and torn leaves. Inner criteria are also valuable; trust what your intuition says when you put your hand on the plant. Any beginner can ask if this is the right plant to take and get an answer. Herbalists find that herbs work better when they ask the plant's permission and guidance before collecting, and give thanks during the process, though the increased medicinal value is difficult to prove in a lab.

The instruction to collect during specific seasons or times of day isn't based on any fanciful idea; guidelines for medicinal harvesting are standardized among traditional herbalists because there are biochemical changes known to affect an herb's therapeutic value. More than once, modern research "proving that plants don't work as claimed" was done on parts collected at the wrong time of year.

Collect herbs in paper or open containers, as plastic bags are an affront to the environment and make the herbs sweat too much. When returning from the field, dry-brush or carefully wash cut plants to remove all dirt and other extraneous material. Since herbs are collected when water levels in the plants are low, it is important not to over-wet them. Avoid roadside collection, as lead, car exhaust, and other pollutants will make the most medicinal herbs into a poisonous cup of tea. Ask permission to pick herbs in organic orchards, wild places that may be on private land, or gardens without pesticides.

Drying

Plants contain a lot of water. One handful of fresh herb is equivalent to about one dried tablespoonful. We dry herbs to use later, though window-box gardens and ceramic pots on kitchen counters make many herbs available year-round. Almost all herbs can be used fresh. The herbs described in this book that are best used fresh are:

- feverfew herb (*Chrysanthemum parthenium*), taken daily to prevent migraines
- shepherd's purse herb (*Capsella bursa-pastoris*), used as an astringent for heavy menstrual, post-partum, or internal bleeding
- cleavers herb (*Galium aparine*), used to improve lymphatic circulation and immune response when lymph nodes are swollen

To dry herbs, cut roots and bulbs in thin slices, like carrots or onions for soup. Cut fleshy leaves (mullein, comfrey) in strips for easier drying at low temperature without the risk of mold growth. The best drying temperature is 105 to 140 degrees F (40 to 60 degrees C) for roots and bark, 85 to 105 degrees F (30 to 40 degrees C) for leaves and flowers. Arrange herbs in single layers (overlapping leaves may turn moldy) on trays, flat baskets, or paper towels, allowing air to circulate. This method minimizes enzyme breakdown and loss of heat-sensitive chemicals.

Drying herbs in the sun is not a good idea; herbs dry quickly, but they lose their color, smell, taste, and therapeutic effects. Shade drying on a dry day works for most herbs if you can leave them spread them out and undisturbed. If you dry herbs outdoors, bring herbs inside at night to protect them from dew. Turn plant parts once or twice a day for even exposure to air.

Deep freezing works if you have the equipment. Food dehydrators work well for the fleshier slices of roots and leaves with hairs (the latter trap moisture and can make drying difficult).

Another drying method for stems with leaves, flowers, or both is to bundle three to five herb stems together and secure them with twine or twist ties (not so good) or small rubber bands (very good). Hang them upside down from a rafter for even airflow, for one to five days.

Herbs must have only eight to ten percent moisture when they are dry, or they will mold. An herb is dry when it snaps or crumbles like a thin cracker. Each herb has its own individual sound when it snaps. The way it breaks is called its *fracture*. The fracture of roots and stems particularly tells the herbalist which plant she has, thanks to the science of *pharmacognosy* (recognizing crude herb material by eye or under microscopes).

Storage

Dry herbs, stored as unbroken as possible, should last at least a full year. Exposed bundles start to lose their value in a month. Crumbled or powdered herbs fit in containers better, but they won't be as potent when you need to use them. Some plant materials, such as oak bark, are so indestructible that they can be stored and used for quite a few years, but until you get to know the peculiarities of the herbs, it's best to use up dried herbs in one year.

This encourages us, in the spring, summer, and fall, to take only what we need for the nongrowing season ahead. By winter's end, new growth out in the fields allows old herbs in the cupboard to be returned to the compost pile or used in a dream pillow mix or potpourri.

We never need as much as we think of some herbs. Start experimenting with one or two ounces of each dried herb, not pounds, unless you have a specific need for more.

The object of herb storage is to keep the herbs from losing their properties to heat, light, air, and contaminants (smoke, air fresheners). The best containers for storing dry herbs are glass jars with tight-fitting lids, tins, or brown paper bags.

Brown paper bags are available and reusable, and they keep herbs dry and protected from light. Large paper bags can hold whole dried herb stems. Paper bags also tie off with long twist-ties or twine and stack away well. If home-dried herbs still contain some moisture, paper bags allow them to breathe and finish drying (any herb that becomes moldy must be composted).

Glass jars are better for protecting herbs in climates that are bug-infested, dry, or extremely moldy. Glass jars are also nicer to look at, but don't leave them in direct sun. Dark glass jars work best.

Preparation

To use herbs, cut them down to workable size. If you purchase herbs, you can buy them whole, cut and sifted, or powdered to various degrees. The only herb discussed frequently in this book that I recommend you buy powdered is wild yam root (*Dioscorea villosa*), as it is too hard on home blenders and coffee grinders.

It is easy to make herbal preparations for internal use or external application. Some preparations are made with the herb and water, some with the herb and oil, and some with the herb and a *menstruum,* which is a fluid that has stronger solvent properties than water (in order from weak to strong: vinegar, glycerin, or alcohol).

Water preparations, whether for internal use (tea) or external use (compress, poultice, wash) only last for one to three days. Preparations made with menstruums last from four months to several years without refrigeration, loss of effect, or spoilage.

Some preparations involve heat: hot water for tea, compresses, and poultices; gently heated vinegar for herbal vinegar tinctures; and gently heated oil for herbal oils. Some preparations do not involve heat: regular alcohol tinctures; cold infusions of mucilage-rich herbs such as marshmallow root; and glycerin extracts.

Herb Teas

Infusions   An infusion is a simple tea made with one or more herbs steeped in boiled water. In Europe, an infusion is called a *tisane*. For lighter plant parts—flowers, leaves, and aromatic parts—it doesn't take much time or heat to get the properties of the plant into the tea.

To make an infusion, weigh out one ounce of dry herbs (one herb or a mixture of herbs, as long as the measured amount is one ounce). Add one pint (two cups) of boiling water to the herbs. Some herbs taste better if you use more than two cups of water, and some—chamomile flowers, for example—are so light and fluffy that it takes more than two cups to cover the herbs.

You will need a medium-to-good-quality kitchen scale to weigh the herbs, and a glass or ceramic teapot to put them in. A clean glass canning jar with a lid works, but recycled juice bottles may crack when hot water is added. Stainless steel is acceptable, but aluminum or plastic containers are not. Unchipped enameled aluminum is fine. The teapot or container should have a good, close-fitting lid.

The aroma should mostly stay in the hot water to go into your body, so if you make a pot of peppermint tea and the whole room smells terrific but the tea has no taste, try a better-fitting lid.

Steep the herbs for ten to twenty minutes; the longer they steep, the more astringent tannins and bitter flavors they will yield, so there is little benefit in steeping them longer. Strain the tea through a bamboo or metal-wire mesh, cloth, or other strainer. Drink the strained herb tea one cup at a time before or between meals, three cups a day, unless different directions for a plant are given.

It is fine to drink herb tea cold if you wish, with a little honey or natural sweetener—never refined sugar or a sugar substitute. Reheating a cup at a time is okay, but don't microwave herbal tea or boil it to death.

There are also cold infusions, which are especially appropriate for herbs rich in heat-sensitive constituents, such as volatile oils (the most aromatic part of herbs) and *mucilages* (slimy starches that are soothing to inflamed tissue). Herbs that have volatile oils include rose petal, peppermint leaf, and lemon balm flower. Mucilaginous herbs include marshmallow root, slippery elm bark, and chia seeds.

Cold infusions are made with the herb and cold water, which are left covered for one to eight hours, depending on how fibrous the plant pieces are and how delicate the plant's chemicals are. The proportions are the same as with hot infusions: one ounce of herb to a pint or more of water.

Decoctions   A *decoction,* from the Latin word meaning "I cook," is an herb tea that is simmered rather than steeped (infused). This process is appropriate for harder plant parts, such as twigs, bark, seeds, and roots, which require the pressure of sustained heat to coax their chemicals out into the tea.

The preparation method is the same: one ounce of dry herb(s) to a pint of water (more than one pint may be used if it helps cover the herbs in the pot). In a saucepan or other heat-safe container, cover the herbs with the water, put the lid in place, and simmer on medium-low heat. The minimum time is ten minutes; the maximum depends on how dense and tough the plant pieces are. The average time for decoction is fifteen to twenty minutes, though you can check by tasting the tea. If it has no flavor after fifteen minutes, let it simmer well-covered for another ten minutes before straining and drinking.

Drink one cup of the tea two to four times a day; the average is three cups a day. You may add honey, lemon, or other flavorings if you wish. However, most herb flavors will grow on you if you let them—and no amount of sweetener will make some bitter herbs taste better. Drink your herbs and chase them with clear water.

Compresses and Poultices

A compress is simply an external application of hot or cold herb liquid. A poultice includes the herb sludge still mixed in with the liquid.

An example of a compress made with tea is a lavender compress, applied over the eyes, forehead, or temples, to relieve a headache. To make a lavender compress, first make a strong infusion, using one to two ounces of lavender flowers to a pint of water, and strain. While the tea is still hot, dip a clean cloth into the tea and wring it out, leaving it slightly wet. Fold and place the cloth over the forehead and eyes for fifteen minutes, refreshing the cloth in the lavender tea as often as necessary to keep the aroma pleasantly strong.

Another example, for bruising, is to decoct witch hazel bark, strain, and let it cool. If needed, add ice or put the tea in the freezer until cold (not frozen). Dip a cloth or towel in and wring it out, then wrap it tightly around a swollen ankle or on a bad bruise to ease swelling and speed the healing. This may be repeated as often as needed. Leave in place a total of forty to sixty minutes at a time; this may be repeated indefinitely.

Compresses of anti-inflammatory and vulnerary herbs reduce facial blemishes (chamomile flowers and cucumber pulp), arthritis (wintergreen herb), and a hundred different external or joint complaints.

A poultice is like a compress, but with the herbs still in the water. A poultice of chickweed herb or oat straw herb will relieve itching. Even a bath with rolled oats in a sock or muslin bag can take the edge off a skin rash or itchy condition.

A "drawing poultice" is made out of equal parts of marshmallow root or leaf, slippery elm bark, and comfrey root, mixed as a ground dried powder with sufficient water to make a wet paste, and placed thickly over an infected wound or splinter. It will act like a vacuum and pull the infection or splinter out from its entry point without scarring the surrounding inflamed tissue.

Capsules

The dried powder of any herb may be put into gelatin capsules to be swallowed. The most common gelatin capsule sizes are #0 and #00. The larger #00 size is often better for home use because it holds about 250 mg (milligrams) of ground herb. This makes a standard daily dose easy to figure out: two #00 capsules hold 500 mg; this dose repeated twice a day (four capsules of 250 mg each) totals 1,000 mg, or one gram of herb per day. A safe, conservative practice is to take two to three capsules at a time, two to three times a day, for a total of four to six capsules (1,000 to 1,500 mg).

Because digestion is often slow when we are ill, the extraction from a gelatin capsule in our stomachs or intestines isn't always as complete as it is with a pot of hot tea or other liquids. The advantage of capsules is convenience. Physical contact between herbs and the digestive tract is especially useful for surfaces lower down that require soothing demulcents (marshmallow root and leaf), anti-inflammatories (licorice root), or astringent, vulnerary (wound-healing) herbs (St. Johnswort herb or calendula flowers). When a larger dose is needed for quick effects, the maximum dose before the digestion starts to rebel from all those capsules and ground dried herbs is about four capsules at a time, six times a day. This is twenty caps a day of 250 mg each, equaling a total of five grams.

The problem with buying any herbal products, especially capsules, is that you have to take the manufacturer's word about the quality of herb inside; you can't smell it or see much of it. Herb quality is important for getting therapeutic effects. Self-help may mean sitting down twice a month for a couple of hours and making your own herbal products. It is very economical.

To create your own herbal capsules, select the herbs by reading the relevant section of this book. If you create your own herbal formula, limit yourself to seven or fewer herbs or there may not be enough of any one herb in the capsule. Use a coffee grinder to powder each herb separately, as some grind down more cooperatively than others.

Mix the powders well in a clean, dry container, using a spoon or a wire whisk. You can scoop two halves of an empty capsule together in the powder to fill the capsules.

A better way to make your own capsules is to buy a simple machine called a Cap-M-Quick; it costs less than fifteen dollars at most herb shops or health food stores, and makes fifty capsules in twenty minutes.

Tinctures

The word *tincture* comes from the Latin word for "tinting" because berries and roots made good dyes and paints in times past. Tinctures are extracts made with alcohol and water; they are appropriate for drawing out plant chemicals that are not soluble in water.

Some plant constituents are water-soluble, and others require stronger solvents such as alcohol. Tinctures extract both types without using heat. The kind of alcohol used is drinkable—never rubbing alcohol or isopropyl alcohol. For home processing, use a liquor that contains at least 40% alcohol (80 proof or higher), such as vodka, brandy, or other spirits. Professional herbalists often use medicinal grain alcohol (almost 96% alcohol), which they dilute to the appropriate strength for each plant. In some states this can be purchased in liquor stores under various brand names such as Ever Clear.

Extracts are similar to tinctures, but they are often five times as concentrated as tinctures, and hence the doses are correspondingly smaller.

Herbalists use tinctures because they are concentrated and convenient. They have a fuller array of medicinal plant chemicals than capsules or tea because the alcohol and water extract more of the whole herb's properties. Tinctures are steeped for two weeks before they are strained and used. Because it is concentrated, a teaspoon of tincture will usually have herbal action equivalent to one cup of tea. Because they are preserved with alcohol, tinctures do not need refrigeration and have a long shelf life.

Tinctures made from fresh plant materials are often full of life, but most tinctures can also be made from dried plants.

Tinctures make a small herb supply go a long way. An ounce of dried herb per day is used in medicinal teas; an ounce of dried herb made into a tincture yields ten days of herbal medicine at a full adult dose of one teaspoonful three times a day. Tinctures also travel well. Though the dose is best taken in a cup of water for quick absorption and an easier time going down, alcohol tinctures can be taken in a moment without any preparation required. When a formula is needed, it is easy to mix two or more single plant tinctures together. Even alcohol and glycerin tinctures can be mixed if the person has no alcohol allergy, addiction, or other sensitivity (such as pregnancy).

Not everyone can tolerate alcohol, and there are many ways to avoid it by using herbs in capsules, teas, and extracts including glycerin tinctures. The average medicinal dose of tincture is one teaspoon of herb vodka or brandy, diluted in one eight-ounce glass of water, taken three times a day. If there is no allergy or alcoholism, this is not enough to do damage to a sick person, especially since a tincture may be taken with food, in smaller doses, or less frequently.

Folk Tinctures   Making tinctures at home is easy and far more economical than buying herb liquids. If you start with good-quality herbs and follow the directions I provide here, your homemade tincture will be as good as anything with a printed label that costs far more.

Place the herbs in a jar, cover them with alcohol, let them sit for two weeks, then strain. We can get fancier, and further instructions follow, but that's basically it. All you need is clean kitchenware and the best herbs you can find. If you make a concentrated herbal tincture from old, dusty, low-grade herbs, you will only have concentrated low-grade herbs.

To make the simplest "folk" tincture for home use, fill a clean, dry jar halfway with dry herb. Sterilized canning jars work well. Cover the herb with medium-quality brandy, vodka, or rum with a 40% or 50% alcohol content (80 or 100 proof). Cheap brands contain impurities and unwanted chemicals; expensive brands are unnecessary since the herb flavor will dominate in the end. If pure grain alcohol is available, use a mixture of 50% water and 50% alcohol.

The liquid (the menstruum) should cover the top of the herbs by about one inch. Close the container with a tight-fitting lid. Shake the jar so that every bit of the herb is moistened. Label it with the plant name and date. Don't even think for a minute that you will remember what this is in two weeks, especially if you make more than one at a time.

Leave the jar in a dark, cool cupboard for at least two weeks. This process, when herbs steep in liquid over time without heat, is called *macerating*. Take the jar out and shake it for five minutes once or twice every day so that all the herb material is equally wet—otherwise, it won't be as fully extracted, resulting in a weaker tincture. After the first few days, some herbs will have soaked up all the liquid and it may be necessary to top off the jar with a few more tablespoons of alcohol to keep the herbs covered. Envision your healing intent for this tincture each time you shake it ("this will help me build dense bones, nourish my uterus, clear my hot flashes").

After two weeks, the tincture is ready to be poured out, but you can leave it indefinitely until you get around to pressing it out. This "pressing out" is more like "wringing out." Place layered cheesecloth, thin unbleached muslin, or other fine-mesh straining cloth in a wire-mesh strainer with a handle, placing these inside a bigger clean mixing bowl or other container. Pour the liquid and herbs into the cloth and strainer (if you made a big batch, do a handful or so of wet herb at a time). Gather up the cloth around the wet herb and wring it between your hands. Use a big enough piece of cloth so that the herb doesn't squish out the sides. "Milk" the liquid downward into the bowl. The strainer is for catching any chunks of herb that fall out of the cloth. The tincture may stain your hands and clothes, so wear clean dishwashing gloves and old clothes.

Pour the strained liquid tincture into a clean, dry, glass bottle with a tight-fitting lid, and label it with the herb name and date. Some sediment will eventually settle on the bottom of the tincture bottle. You can leave it in, or you can remove it by pouring the clear liquid carefully off the top; this is called *decanting*. If the glass is clear or light-colored, keep the tincture out of direct light, and store it away from heat.

Tinctures for Clinical Use   The practice of making tinctures can be much more exact than the method just described. Tinctures for clinical use have a measured amount of herb and a measured amount of liquid. A tincture that is "1:5 60%" has one part of the herb weighed out, extracted in five parts of liquid, and that liquid is 60% alcohol. The simple rule is: to every ounce of dry herb, add five fluid ounces of menstruum for a one in five (1:5) concentration of herb to liquid. To two ounces of herb, add ten fluid ounces of liquid. For four ounces of herb, add twenty fluid ounces of menstruum.

Herbalists know from experience and modern testing methods which herbs extract best with a low percentage of alcohol (for example, marshmallow because of its mucopolysaccharides) and which require pure grain spirits (myrrh, because of its water-resistant resin). The lowest alcohol concentration for good preservative purposes is about 18%, and a safer number, allowing for human error and variations in herb batches is 25%.

The mildest menstruum of 25% alcohol (75% water) is best for herbs that would make a good cup of tea as an infusion: demulcent herbs with mucilage (marshmallow root and leaf, plantain leaf), aromatic herbs containing volatile oils, and herbs of light weight (peppermint leaf, chamomile flower), or whose constituents yield easily to water (tannins, some glycosides).

The next group of herbs, requiring 45%-alcohol menstruums, are volatile oil-containing herbs from denser plant parts (aniseed, valerian root), and herbs with both chemicals that come out in water (55% water in this menstruum) and chemicals that need to be extracted and preserved in more than 25% alcohol.

For the third group of herbs that have water-soluble constituents but even more non-water-soluble constituents, we mix 40% water with 60% alcohol. The British Herbal Pharmacopoeia (BHP) has an additional category with a 70% alcohol menstruum. In my practice, I have divided the herbs made with 70% between my 60% menstruum and the undiluted 96% menstruums. The BHP doesn't use a 25% low-alcohol menstruum, which is useful.

A fourth group, using undiluted grain alcohol (approximately 96%), is for tough plant material. For instance, myrrh resin will steep in a cup of just-boiled water forever without giving up much of its antimicrobial properties to the water. Not even 60% alcohol will get much out of myrrh. But with 90% alcohol, myrrh tincture will slay hordes of invading bacteria.

Fresh Plant Tinctures   Many herbalists find the essence or living qualities of the plants important to healing, but fresh plant tinctures are apt to spoil if made by the methods I have so far described. There are two easy guidelines for making fresh herb tinctures: don't add water to the alcohol menstruum, and use one part of fresh herb to two parts of menstruum. Whether an herb is fleshy and wet, like comfrey root, or fairly dry to the touch, like horsetail leaves or rosemary leaves and flowers, the water in the herb is considered to be enough for the water portion of the menstruum. Picking the herbs on a dry mid-morning in the right season helps, as does letting them wilt a little (up to a few hours) so that there is less water in the tincture.

The menstruum for fresh plant tinctures should be 100% alcohol, but if all you have is 150 proof (75% alcohol) or 180 proof (90% alcohol) grain alcohol, that will work just fine.

Fresh plants may be tinctured this same way in undiluted glycerin instead of alcohol (see "Glycerin Tinctures," following). They macerate for two weeks and shouldn't spoil or need refrigeration, but with fresh plants it is always wise to make small batches at first and check them often. If a batch is moldy, there was too much water. Don't try to save it; dilute it with water and compost it. Then begin again.

Vinegar Tinctures   Vinegar is adequate, but not terrific, as a solvent or preservative (it is stronger than water, but weaker than glycerin or alcohol). It is most useful for herbs that contain alkaloids, such as lobelia. Herbs that are tinctured in vinegar have a shelf life of about two to six months in the refrigerator. Be aware that vinegar, like oil, ruins the inside of canning jar lids after a while, so replace them often as needed. Vinegar does have health-promoting properties, with its stimulation of gastric juices and mineral absorption. It isn't viable for some people, however, if they are allergic to vinegar, dislike the taste, or need stronger herbal effects than many vinegar tinctures can give.

If this method of tincturing is your choice, use only raw (unheated) apple cider vinegar, since you'll have to heat it once yourself and heat isn't good for vinegar. It is best to use dry herb; fresh herb in vinegar spoils easily since the water in the herb dilutes a weak preservative even more.

Whether you use the folk method (cover the herb with an inch or so of menstruum) or measure for more exact tinctures, heat the vinegar to below boiling. Pour it over the herb in a clean, dry jar. Store it away from heat and light for two weeks and shake it daily, as with the alcohol tinctures described above. After pressing the vinegar tincture out of the herb, repeat with a new batch of dried herb for stronger tinctures.

Glycerin Tinctures   Another way to avoid alcohol in tinctures is to use glycerin, creating what are called *glycerides, glycerites,* or glycerine tinctures. These are made the same way as alcohol tinctures, but using glycerin for the menstruum. Glycerin is a better solvent for plant chemicals than water or vinegar, but it isn't as strong as alcohol, so glycerin tinctures will be slightly weaker than alcohol tinctures.

There is an advantage to using glycerin when combining herbs that are rich in tannins with herbs that are rich in alkaloids. In alcohol tinctures, tannins and alkaloids bind together, making the herb(s) less effective. Glycerin prevents this binding, or precipitation, of alkaloids and tannins, keeping them suspended in solution.

For dried herb tinctures in glycerin, always use a menstruum of 60% glycerin and 40% water. Less glycerin tends to make a moldy tincture. Use vegetable glycerin instead of animal glycerin, available at natural food stores and mail-order herb suppliers. The cost of glycerin is similar to that of alcohol.

One advantage of a glycerin tincture is that it makes bitter herbs more palatable, which can be especially useful for children and sensitive people. Glycerin tastes sweet without having the negative effects on blood-sugar level associated with honey or sugar. However, diabetics who use herbs extracted in glycerin should watch their blood glucose to make sure it remains at the proper level.

For fresh plant glycerin tinctures, the water content already in the fresh herb material is considered the water portion of the menstruum. Use full-strength, undiluted glycerin to make tinctures from fresh plants. The weight proportions of plant material to glycerin menstruum is 1:2, meaning one ounce of fresh herb is covered with two fluid ounces of undiluted glycerin. Some herbs won't fit in this small a volume of liquid, so they have to be finely chopped.

Herb Juice and Herb Honey

Herbs can also be juiced, though herb juices have no shelf life and must be consumed on the spot to prevent loss of properties from enzymatic degradation. Juices may be preserved with alcohol: three parts of juice to one part of undiluted (95 to 96%) alcohol. Let the juice sit for two days. The finished product is about 22% alcohol and will last at least one year without refrigeration.

Herbs may be extracted in honey—especially aromatic herbs such as thyme, sage, or ginger—to treat sore throats and nausea due to blood sugar changes. Onion and garlic honeys make an excellent cold, flu, and respiratory ailment remedy. Thinly slice raw garlic or onion (or both), and pack the slices well in a clean jar until it is three-fourths full; cover with unheated raw honey and close the lid (glass jars with rubber seals and a glass lid on a hinge work well). Let sit for one to four hours or overnight; take one tablespoon every half hour as needed for up to three days, or take a teaspoon daily for prevention and immune-system maintenance. Store the extraction in the refrigerator, where it will keep for at least six weeks.

Oils

Herbal oils are useful lubricants and healing agents. Rice bran, almond, hazelnut, and sesame oils are the lightest and best-absorbed oils for skin and vaginal lubrication because they soak in so quickly. Unheated green olive oil doesn't soak in as quickly, but the less filtered and more green it is, the more earthy the smell will be and the more chlorophyll it will contain (chlorophyll has many healing attributes). It's good for reducing inappropriate organisms in the intestines, improving oxygen in the blood, and reducing gas.

Herbal oils (St. Johnswort, calendula, comfrey, or wild yam) can be used daily and during intercourse as needed, for lubrication and healing. To make these herbal oils, placed four ounces *total* of one or more of the above-mentioned dried herbs in a clean, dry quart jar, and cover them with green, unfiltered olive oil, sesame oil, almond oil, or other vegetable oil. One inch of oil should be seen above the level of herb in the jar. With a tight-fitting lid in place, put the jar in a saucepan of water and keep it on low heat for three days.

If you will not be around to prevent accidents, another way to make herbal oil is to leave the jar in a warm place (the top of a refrigerator or water heater) or in the sun for ten days. The usual precautions against storing herb preparations in the heat and light don't apply here, since it is the low heat over time that draws the herb's properties into the oil. Be sure not to get the oil so hot that it turns rancid. At the end of three to ten days, when the oil has turned the color of the herb, strain the herb out through muslin or cheesecloth.

Herb Salves   Return ¼ cup of the filtered herb oil to a clean, dry saucepan and add 1 tablespoon of coconut butter or cocoa butter; melt over low heat. Test the consistency by periodically placing a spoonful of the mixture in the refrigerator for a few minutes to see how solid it gets upon cooling (use a clean spoon each time). If the herbal salve is too soupy, add more coconut or cocoa butter, or melt in one or more walnut-sized pieces of beeswax. Pour the salve into a clean, dry jar with a tight-fitting lid, and label it. The natural preservatives in some herbs will keep them from needing refrigeration, but use the salve up within the year.

Be aware that oils ruin the rubber seals on canning jars after a while; use a plastic bag around the lid and ring, and it will still screw down airtight. Oil-based preparations are not ideal when yeast or fungal infections are present. Moisture and heat are sealed in by oils and ointments, making yeasts too comfortable. In healthy people, the antimicrobial qualities of the herbal oils make them less of a problem than plain vegetable oils, and even helpful in fighting fungal or yeast infections. If the problem worsens with their use, however, please see more therapeutic herbs for candida in Chapter 19.

St. Johnswort oil is a red color, and acts as an anti-inflammatory lubricant. Calendula oil is golden, and is especially good for healing small tears or abrasions of vaginal mucosa. Both are antiviral, though the extent of this property in oil used locally is variable. Wild yam oil is the basis for many natural creams used in menopause, improving vaginal lubrication and healing.

Castor oil is made from the castor bean plant, also called *Palma Christi*. The external use of castor oil is usually as a hot compress to reduce swellings and overgrowths of fibrous tissue or mixed cellular growths. It is available at herb shops, natural food stores, some drugstores, and from suppliers listed in the Appendix.

To use castor oil, heat at least 4 ounces in a small saucepan or in a double-boiler. Be careful about spills to avoid burns or grease fires. Pour oil into the center of a large piece of flannel (usually hand-towel-size) and fold over once or twice to hold oil (now mostly soaked into flannel). Add more oil as needed to saturate the material. Place the hot oily towel on the skin over any bruise, swelling, or growth. This might be over the abdomen, pelvis, or breast and surrounding lymph nodes.

Reheat the towel or flannel by redipping it in the pan of warmed castor oil, whenever the application gets cool. Hot water bottles over another clean, dry towel placed on top of the oil-soaked flannel help keep the warmth in. Hot water bottles are better than heating pads because they are easier to clean up, and the electromagnetic pulse of the heating pad has a negative effect on the body. Leave castor oil in place for twenty minutes to an hour, as long as it is hot; hot water bottles can be refilled as needed. It isn't recommended to reheat the oily towel, although you can add new heated castor oil to the flannel or towel. This is worth the stained towels and cleanup.

Since castor oil is used externally to break down growths or lumps for elimination, help your body's general elimination. Eat light, healthy meals so that the breakdown of tissue does not proceed faster than the body's ability to safely eliminate what is being stirred back into general circulation. Repeat the castor oil compress twice a week for seven weeks or even daily for three weeks. Quicker results from more frequent use may be seen, but this requires more rest and superb nutrition and elimination. Otherwise, if the body is under normal stress and must eliminate toxins eaten in a standard diet, it will be breaking up stubborn growths such as fibroids inside faster than it can tolerate or eliminate. Proceeding in a relaxed way rather than a rapid way is recommended anyway, because healing can be tiring.

Adding therapeutic essential oils such as geranium, marjoram, clary sage, or lavender (not perfume scents) to the castor oil is helpful when stress and a depressed self-image accompany any health condition. Do not add these essential oils to the castor oil while it is heating, or the essential (volatile) oils will evaporate; stir them into the castor oil just before pouring it into the flannel or towel. The aromatherapy value of the essential oils is experienced by most women as uplifting to the spirits, but they also penetrate through the skin to aid castor oil in reducing inflammation. For every 3 to 4 ounces of castor oil, add 15 to 20 drops of the pure essential oils of your choice (available at herb/natural food stores or by mail order). It does take a little effort to be consistent, but a difference may be noticed in just two to eight weeks.

PART TWO

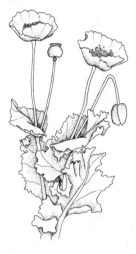

Problems of Menses

3

Amenorrhea: A Lack of Menstrual Cycles

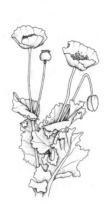

Definition

Amenorrhea is simply the absence of a menstrual period. What isn't so simple is determining the cause. There are several possible causes, and not all cases require treatment. For instance, one of the most common causes for a missed menstrual cycle is lack of rest, for which the treatment is to do a lot of nothing. Amenorrhea is normal before puberty, during pregnancy, during breast-feeding (lactation), and after menopause.

Symptoms and Signs

The description and the symptoms are the same: a missed period for three months in a row without any obvious cause, such as pregnancy. Because there are so many interrelated causes of amenorrhea, any other symptoms that occur will vary.

Cause

Amenorrhea is called "primary" before puberty, and this is not usually a condition that requires treatment. Normally *menarche,* the onset of menstruation, occurs any time between the ages of eight and eighteen. These first periods may occur without ovulation. Amenorrhea before age seventeen is only of concern when it signals other hormonal imbalances or congenital problems, identified by a physician.

"Secondary" amenorrhea refers to periods that stop for some reason after they have started. This is what most people mean when they refer to amenorrhea. The difference between amenorrhea and a missed period or irregular cycle is that, in amenorrhea, at least three months in a row go by without menstrual bleeding. The causes of secondary amenorrhea are as diverse as diabetes, thyroid deficiency, depression, and sometimes even tumors.

The following reasons for why one may miss a period will help women determine what manner of attention their body is requesting.

Amenorrhea does not always indicate pathology. Normally, menstruation occurs about two weeks after the release of an egg, unless a woman becomes pregnant. When women are not feeling well, they might not have the extra juice for that perfect dance of hormones that causes an egg to be released. The body knows that times of ill health or extreme stress are not good times to start a new life to form, should fertilization occur. Furthermore, if there is no fertilization, the body may not be able to afford the energy lost in menstrual blood after ovulation. But if being stressed out and tired were always enough to throw our hormones off to this degree, we wouldn't have nearly as many people on the planet as we do; being tired is not good birth control.

Pregnancy is another common cause for a missed period, and this must be ruled out before using any herbs to bring on a normal menstrual flow.

A third cause of amenorrhea is travel, especially through time zones or by air, as women's biological rhythms undergo shifts. Travel is often associated with loss of sleep, excitement, and possibly illness or even malnutrition. But travel and fatigue are not diseases, and these activities do not automatically cause amenorrhea.

Malnutrition due to a stressful life, abnormal weight (obesity or low body weight), poverty, isolation, or inadequate cooking facilities can also cause amenorrhea. Malnutrition exists among affluent, educated women as well as the growing number of women at the poverty level. In my practice, I see women who cannot menstruate because they are so empty from eating little more than raw sprouts while holding down a demanding job.

Amenorrhea can also result from training for a marathon or exercising obsessively more than a few hours a day. Sometimes intelligent young women with painful backgrounds ask me for herbs to fix their irregular cycles. This is to be done, of course, while they go through abuse counseling and start new love relationships.

Do these women without periods need strong hormonal herbs for this crisis? No. This is the time to give them the mildest reproductive tonics and herbs to nourish their depleted systems, followed by safe nervine relaxants or calming medicinal plants. The herbalist has a dual responsibility to respect a request for herbs to kick-start normal periods, as well as to use herbs safely for long-term health.

Anorexia nervosa and other eating disorders including overeating are an increasingly common cause of amenorrhea, requiring professional counseling and support.

If a woman chooses to take the Herbal Formula II described later in this chapter, it may help and cannot hurt, but it won't start periods in a woman who isn't eating.

Conventional Medical Care

The medical view, which does not usually respect women's wisdom, says that when we miss a period for three months for any reason other than pre-puberty, pregnancy, lactation, or menopause, we may be suffering from a disease. While it is true that we may require attention, this could be loving attention to oneself instead of medical intervention. Conventional treatment depends on the cause. It may include giving progesterone to see if a functioning uterus can be kick-started into menstruation.

Herbal Treatment

The objective of holistic herbalism is to work on functional disturbances rather than on pathology. We look for simple causes that affect our normal functioning, instead of immediately suspecting the worst and looking for disease. Herbs have a tremendous success rate in balancing hormones, relieving pelvic congestion, and integrating nerve and hormone signals. This herbal approach for amenorrhea is straightforward in the absence of organic disease diagnosed by a physician or pregnancy.

Emmenagogues such as *Achillea* (yarrow flower) bring on normal menstruation by optimizing more than one body function. Usually this broad-based natural approach is powerfully healing. Occasionally this is not enough. Whatever state of health or disease women are starting from, the herbs described in this chapter aim at a balance of reproductive hormonal and menstrual cycles.

As you have seen, many forms of amenorrhea have their origins in stress. But what can a stressed-out person do? The herbs that help us find inner peace are not the strongest tranquilizers. Mildly calming plants, such as *Scutellaria* (skullcap herb) or *Passiflora* (passionflower herb), taken during a crisis can reduce the immediate feeling of frazzled nerves. Taking the pressure off may be enough to allow a menstrual cycle to reestablish its natural rhythm.

Other herbal remedies build up a woman's ability to withstand life's pressures. These herbs are called adaptogens. An example of an adaptogenic herb is Siberian ginseng. Research based on long-term, large-scale, voluntary human trials on factory workers in Siberia showed that Siberian ginseng benefits people who are under ongoing stress.

Let's look at stress for a moment. Stress initially puts the body in a state of "alarm," which is eventually replaced by adaptation, and finally gives way to exhaustion. In the alarm stage, a surge of adrenaline prepares us for fight or flight. This stage involves a co-activation of all the nerves and endocrine glands involved in the stress response. Oxygen goes to the brain and we think more rapidly for the moment; blood sugar rushes into our muscles to make us stronger than we usually feel. Many people love the adrenaline rush; feeling brighter and stronger becomes habit-forming, so one may not want to stop the stressful stimuli.

There are better ways for women to stay bright and strong, and herbs can help undo an unhealthy addiction to these hormones. But, more importantly, we can use herbs such as *Ginkgo* (ginkgo leaf) to improve the way our brains get more oxygen, even without stress. We can improve blood-sugar balance with bitters such as *Taraxacum* (dandelion root) and mild endocrine tonics such as *Vaccinium* (blueberry leaf). Women can optimize circulation to muscles and internal organs with *Rosmarinus* (rosemary leaf). Finally, we can use adaptogenic herbs such as Siberian ginseng to nourish and heal our nerves and endocrine glands, including the adrenal glands, which take the worst beating in our nonstop response to stress. If we're going to heal the earth, we'll need our strength. Let the earth lend you some of hers.

The underlying causes of amenorrhea can be addressed effectively so that the symptoms clear as a woman's body returns to health. A woman interested in helping herself to heal must take time out to determine what is causing her amenorrhea.

Herbal Formula I, which follows, is designed to relax with one or more relaxing nervines, rebuild with one or more nutritives, balance with tonics for the reproductive system, and warm or energize with circulatory normalizers. The combination of herbs allows menstruation to return, with all its normal physiological controls. It is well-suited to weakened people or those who don't eat right, and it gradually builds up normal body functions.

Herbal Formula I

Urtica dioca (nettle leaf)	1½ ounces
Passiflora incarnata (passionflower leaf)	2 ounces
Angelica archangelica (angelica root)	2 ounces
Achillea millefolium (yarrow leaf/flower)	2 ounces
Rosa canina (rose hips)	2–4 ounces, to taste
Zingiber officinale (ginger root)	½ ounce, to taste

Stir all the dry herbs together in a clean, dry mixing bowl before storing in a tea tin, glass jar, or other container.

Pour 3 cups of boiling water over 1 ounce of the herb mixture in a teapot or glass container; steep fifteen minutes. Drink ½ to 1 cup of tea, two to three times every day, for ten days.

You may save yourself time by making up a big batch of tea to last two or three days; keep it strained and stored in the refrigerator in a glass container with a lid. Leaving the herbs in the tea longer makes it more bitter, but not necessarily better for you. If you can't get one of the herbs, make the combination anyway. Chamomile makes a good substitute here for passionflower. Hibiscus can replace rose hips.

Herbal Formula II is stronger than Herbal Formula I, and has more to offer women who are under a heavier load of stress.

Herbal Formula II

Artemisia vulgaris (mugwort leaf)	1 ounce
Leonurus cardiaca (motherwort leaf/flower)	2 ounces
Mentha piperita (peppermint leaf)	4 ounces
Eleutherococcus senticosus (Siberian ginseng)	2 ounces
Scutellaria lateriflora (skullcap leaf/flower)	3 ounces
Glycyrrhiza glabra (licorice root)	2 ounces

Leave out the mugwort if there is a possibility that you are pregnant. Licorice is a great antiviral and anti-inflammatory remedy that simultaneously soothes your insides and stimulates your liver and adrenal glands. However, if you have high blood pressure, a history of kidney failure, or a problem maintaining your potassium levels, replace the licorice with two ounces of Siberian ginseng root plus one ounce each of marshmallow root and burdock root.

Steep 1 ounce of the herbal mixture in 3 cups of water for ten to fifteen minutes according to the standard instructions in Chapter 2. Drink one cup three times a day for ten to twelve days, then take a one-week break. If no period occurs in that time, drink a weaker tea using only one-half ounce of herb mixture in 3 cups of water every day for another twelve days. It is safe to repeat this dose until a period starts, for up to three months. If you still don't menstruate, you should see a qualified health care provider or herbalist.

Amenorrhea After Taking the Birth Control Pill

Irregular or missed periods often follow the use of synthetic hormones such as the birth control pill. In such a case, add two ounces of *Vitex* (chasteberry) to Herbal Formula I, and drink it as described for a minimum of three months.

Early Menopause

If poor health is contributing to a mature woman's amenorrhea, yet she feels she is not ready for menopause, encouraging results may come from a focus on sound nutrition and emotional well-being. Herbal therapies described in the chapter on menopause (Chapter 23) will help a woman's cycle to continue to its natural end. Herbs cannot force an unnaturally long reproductive life or prevent the inevitable transition through menopause. However, herbal therapy can prolong or even restart cycles if a mature woman's body is capable of maintaining menses in health. "Natural" menopause means augmenting what is healthiest in each woman's nature, not medicating her "just in case." Please see Chapter 23: Menopause for more information.

Nutrition

There is no single eating plan or list of suggested supplements that fits every woman with amenorrhea. Balance of body weight is far more important than taking supplements. When healthy fats are eaten in moderation they help our balance of estrogen and progesterone. Besides eating less processed foods, women can help balance their cycles by eating whole foods on a regular basis. Soy beans, lentils with brown rice, or a slice of organic avocado in a dark green leafy salad are healing, because the small amount of fat is of a higher quality. The body knows how to use these types of fats.

Other Points

Menstrual periods, or a lack of them, are the way our subconscious expresses our connection with life. Choosing a loving world does more good for your health than taking synthetic hormones to force your ovaries to pump out eggs like clockwork or to start a period.

4

PMS: Premenstrual Syndrome

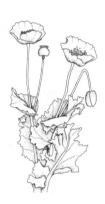

Definition

Premenstrual syndrome (PMS) has over 150 recognized signs and symptoms. What most people think of as PMS are the characteristic emotional changes, particularly anxiety and irritability. There may also be water retention (including breast tenderness), food cravings, depression, digestive changes, skin problems, and a lower pain threshold.

Though premenstrual syndrome and painful periods *(dysmenorrhea)* are not the same, they often go together. Some of the self-help information in this chapter applies to the chapter on dysmenorrhea as well, but I have tried to keep repetition to a minimum.

The symptoms of PMS vary depending on a woman's general health, especially her reproductive history. A woman's hormonal balance can be affected by emotional shock, cultural conditioning, family medical history, nutritional patterns, and self-image.

We are more sensitive premenstrually. When our cervix opens to release the inside of our womb, we are literally more "open." We shed a lining that could have cushioned another life. This is the best time of the month to have visions. Nature's design is for menstruating women to go away, tune in to the messages of their bodies, and reflect on life under the sensitizing influence of lunar tides.

Symptoms and Signs

The recognized symptoms of PMS are grouped into six major patterns or types, identified by a predominant symptom:

- anxiety (Type A)
- craving (Type C)
- depression (Type D)
- hyperhydration (water retention; Type H)
- pain (Type P)
- skin problems (Type S)

A woman might not fit neatly into one of these patterns, but reviewing them can provide insight. In addition to the most common symptoms, other problems linked with PMS include painful cramps, heavy flow, mood swings, hostility, migraines, dizziness, weight gain, allergies, depressed immune-system response, urinary tract problems, and asthma.

Type A: Anxiety and Emotional Changes

Eighty percent of women with PMS have this symptom pattern, characterized by elevated estrogen and low progesterone levels, irritability, nervous tension, mood swings, and water retention, including breast tenderness.

PMS characterized by anxiety could be caused at the level of either the pituitary gland or the ovaries. The best treatment results come from cleansing the liver using hepatic herbs between menses and ovulation. In addition, it helps to decrease intake of caffeine, hot spices, and preservatives.

Type C: Food Cravings

Type C PMS is characterized by a sudden strong appetite, especially for refined carbohydrates. This woman has hypoglycemia, fatigue, and low levels of magnesium in her red blood cells.

Type D: Depression

This type of PMS is characterized by emotional lows, confusion, forgetfulness, being accident-prone, or being easily moved to tears. This PMS pattern often coexists with anxiety and rage. Women may become suicidal. Women who have depression before bleeding may have too much progesterone.

Type H: Hyperhydration

Water retention is sometimes caused by high levels of aldosterone, an adrenal hormone. Water retention with PMS may also be due to stress or high estrogen levels, usually accompanied by a deficiency of magnesium or even dopamine (a neuro-transmitter in the brain).

Type P: Pain

This category of PMS is characterized by a lowered pain threshold and significant muscle aches. Like Type A, and Type S, this form of PMS is made worse by the prostaglandins we make when we eat too much animal protein.

Type S: Skin Problems

A sixth category of PMS is characterized by acne due to high levels of androgens during periods of stress. This overdrive eventually results in chronic adrenal deficiency, made worse by consuming animal fats and dairy products.

Cause

PMS symptoms are noticeably increased during the full moon. Remembering that we are not separate from nature is itself profoundly healing. Just as all the waters of the planet respond to lunar ebb and flow, so do the waters of our bodies. We become "lunatics" only when we deny the pull toward the moonlight. Herbs that help us harmonize this ebb and flow coevolved on this watery body of earth. They give us serenity in fractured times. They are exhilarating and rejuvenating.

Before I describe herbal solutions for PMS, let's take a broader look at what this phenomenon represents. Is the flare-up of emotions and related symptoms triggered by our hormones, or might it be a result of our attempt to adapt to an unresponsive culture?

Women tend to be peacemakers, inviting harmony in professional, social, and domestic settings. Most of the month, we smile and get our own work done, give praise in appreciation of others, and handle little distractions or annoyances with some humor and perspective. But premenstrually, when we have asked someone to feed the dog every day for four days in a row, yet we find ourselves feeding the dog after another long workday, we may speak less than appreciatively. We have other things we must attend to. Our hormones are demanding our attention. We have been pushed by the physiological changes in our bodies to turn inward and take care of ourselves. Stating our preferences may come out in strong words, but to the defensive dog owner we will be guilty as charged: nagging "because of PMS."

Will women need to yell less if herbs help carve out a week of inner peace? Will hormonal calm give us enough distance to ask for the things we need in a more effective way than yelling? Will these improvements encourage others nearest us to give the honor we are due? One can always hope.

But if society respected women's need to withdraw for one day to one week per month, we wouldn't have an epidemic syndrome with 150 known signs and symptoms. In earlier times, when people lived closer to the earth, women's physiology was under the regular influence of moonlight and sunlight. When women bled, they would leave the community for a few days. Often they went to a special cave or a "moon hut" in the woods built of willow. Women lay on their backs and relaxed, looking at the cozy fire that was being tended for them, having their lower abdomens massaged with healing herbal liniments. Post-menopausal women would know which herb teas to give the menstruating women to lighten their mood or bring on a dreamy sleep, what brews to give them for cramps, or how to hold a heated rock to the abdomen, letting the pleasant weight press down and relieve pain when the bleeding began.

If you can't get away to a moon hut, change what you can to get the support that will mean the most to you. For a start, cut yourself a little slack, set aside some time to be by yourself in nature—and take a thermos of healing herb tea with you to work for a week.

Conventional Medical Care

The conventional treatment for PMS ranges from reassurance to antidepressants, and is aimed at reducing symptoms. Women are prescribed tranquilizers, sedatives, birth control pills, or other synthetic forms of progesterone such as Provera, Depo-Provera, or Norgestrel. Medical doctors may also recommend multivitamins or prostaglandin inhibitors such as NSAIDs (nonsteroidal anti-inflammatory drugs, such as aspirin).

Herbal Treatment

The holistic approach to PMS takes into account a woman's medical history and a wider view of her relationships. The treatment may work on several levels at once. There are herbs to take for serenity in the short term while we explore and treat the underlying causes of PMS.

The objective of herbal treatment is to normalize the entire hormonal cycle, starting with the functioning of the *corpus luteum*. This is what we call an ovarian follicle after it releases an egg and begins to produce the hormone *progesterone*. But the use of hormonal herbs is not solely focused on hormone levels or getting rid of the symptoms.

The objective for relieving PMS is to address the woman's entire "wheel" of health factors. The spokes of that wheel vary from woman to woman, but they usually include: diet, state of the nerves, hormone levels, liver function, social conditioning, and general vitality. In this context, improving corpus luteum function may help prevent future PMS episodes, even when life's inevitable stresses rise and fall again. The herbal formula for relieving PMS requires some flexibility, based on treating the woman, not her PMS. I will give you examples of ways to alter the formula depending on the symptoms and circumstances.

Lifestyle Support for Your Herbal Treatment

In addition to herbs, the cure for PMS includes honoring our increased natural sensitivity before each period. The cure means optimizing our health, including our attitude. The cure involves choosing our surroundings carefully. Turn off the blaring, boring TV. It has not earned your loyalty and cannot help you now. Stay quietly by a favorite window or picture for a spell. Just sit. There may be a warm fire to help focus your mind on nothing at all, or perhaps there is just a well-placed candle. Close the open windows of your personality and find yourself.

Sacred time alone, as defined by each woman for herself, is the true treatment for PMS. Women can have time alone without losing jobs or abandoning families, but they will need to sacrifice a few activities somewhere. Sacrifice doesn't mean giving up; it means choosing when to make a sacred gift of something dear, to get back something just as precious.

Herbs are able to change our consciousness so we may change our experience. We have no need to suppress raging hormones or smother bad tempers. The herbs that calm our minds and relax our bodies give us an introspective holiday each month. These plants can change our bodies into "purified temples" where the rhythms of moonlight shine with meaning for us.

Anger, a familiar emotion during PMS, depresses liver function. The idea of anger being stuffed down is easy for everyone to understand as a possible cause of blocked energy. This may result in PMS symptoms including headaches, bloating, or rage. Three areas in the body that tend to get blocked most whenever energy gets stuck are the pelvis (menstrual cramps and pain), chest and breasts (swelling, tenderness, lumps, allergies, and asthma), and throat. This last area points to depressed immunity. If disharmony is established at the gateway to the body, women tend to get more sore throats, colds, or flu around the menses. The reason herbalists treat the liver in PMS is to improve elimination, especially of excess estrogens. Unopposed estrogen may be the most important imbalance herbs can address successfully. For all these reasons, the PMS formulas I describe in this chapter contain herbs that support liver and immune-system function.

Herbs and Time

Some people complain that herbal therapy works too slowly. Our culture wants a tablet and wants it to work *now*. Sometimes herbs work well this way, and sometimes not. But most medicinal herbs do not bring their healing gifts to our bodies as instant fixes. Herbs occur in our biosphere not as concentrated, standardized tablets, but as flavorful, colorful, stimulating, calming, or balancing whole plants.

Taking time for healing disrupts economic or other imposed timetables. But time is the magic ingredient for healing diseases of mismanaged time here in the everyday world. PMS is such a disease.

In earlier civilizations, sick people were given two days to six weeks or more for complete attention to resolving the matter at hand. It is no wonder that herbs, visions, and fasting by sacred pools brought tales of miracle cures down to us through time. Today, we are not always able to take time off. Single mothers, nurses, women under stress, women on night shifts—these are the women I see most often with PMS.

Though it may not seem so, we are able to find time for ourselves within our schedules. Time and space are only human concepts, and we can start conceiving of them differently to create our own real time and space. It's not so hard; the simpler the attitude adjustment the greater may be the effect.

Breathe in and let your mind clear for a moment. Even taking a few deep breaths is physiologically calming. Your body experiences space. Time becomes elastic. A moment of clear-minded deep breathing is as refreshing as a catnap, which is also recommended whenever practical. Breathe out and smile for no particular reason, for no one but yourself. When we smile, our face muscles get a break from the tension stored from jaw to shoulder. When our brain feels even a brief reprieve from stress, it rewards us with brain chemistry changes that help us keep on smiling. It is not necessary to postpone taking time for yourself until all personal and global problems are resolved! Just start where you are. Bigger issues can shift only when we have the breathing space to view them in a new way.

Attitude adjustment thanks to herbs can change PMS into a blessed time for reflection. To be at peace with what *is* brings health closer no matter where each of us stands right now. The natural remedies I describe in this chapter can encourage this sense of peace even before PMS symptoms disappear.

Herbal Formula

Vitex agnus-castus (vitex or chasteberry seed)	2 ounces
Scutellaria lateriflora (skullcap herb)	1 ounce
Smilax ornata (sarsaparilla root)	1 ounce
Taraxacum officinale (dandelion root and leaf)	1 ounce of each

If blood sugar fluctuation and/or fatigue worsen, add:

Eleutherococcus senticosus (Siberian ginseng)	1 ounce
Oplopanax horridum (devil's club root bark)	1 ounce

Don't confuse devil's club with the anti-inflammatory herb devil's claw, often taken by people with arthritis. Devil's club works on food cravings and stress patterns, and helps normalize appetite and blood sugar. With the adaptogenic Siberian ginseng, increased energy feels smooth, not "jumpy."

If stress worsens PMS symptoms, add:

Valeriana officinalis (Valerian root)	1 ounce

Substitute passionflower or Siberian ginseng if you are sensitive to valerian.

If tension or headaches occur with PMS, add:

Lavandula spp. (Lavender flower)	1 ounce

Lavender makes an excellent glycerin tincture. Take ½ to 2 teaspoons diluted in water, herb tea, or juice, as often as needed.

If PMS is worsened by water retention, add:

Taraxacum officinalis (dandelion leaf)	1 ounce
Achillea millefolium (yarrow flower)	½ ounce

Also add one bunch of fresh parsley to your daily diet for two to four days before menses; it is even more effective if taken a few days before water retention begins to build up. Avoid both yarrow and parsley if there is a possibility of pregnancy.

If PMS is made worse simply by expecting painful cramping, refer to Chapter 5: Dysmenorrhea and Chapter 6: Menorrhagia, or add to the formula above:

Viburnum prunifolium (black haw bark)	1 ounce
Viburnum opulus (cramp bark)	2 ounces

Tinctures of either or both of these, or a separate tea, may be taken as needed, one cup of tea or one teaspoon of tincture per dose. This dose may be taken hourly if needed, but limit tincture intake to ten teaspoons over the course of one day. It usually only takes two to three doses to relieve pain, and is especially useful at night.

If migraine headaches occur before or with menses, add to the formula and take the whole formula throughout the month for a minimum of three months:

Chrysanthemum parthenium (feverfew fresh herb extract)   1 ounce

Note that feverfew is usually thought most effective as fresh leaf or fresh plant extract, not tea from dried herb or dried herb in capsules. Freeze-dried herb capsules work for some, but not for others. Feverfew in any form is only occasionally effective in ridding one of a headache once it has begun. Feverfew works best when used throughout the month as a preventive measure; it increases in effectiveness the longer it is used. The fresh herb is also used, though its leaf is bitter to the taste and one possible side effect of chewing it is mouth blisters. If you can correctly identify this herb (it can be confused with others), eat one leaf per day. If you are one of the unlucky few who get blisters, discontinue; after three days try fresh plant extract instead, which does not seem to cause this problem.

If either skin problems or constipation accompany PMS, add:

Rumex crispus (yellow dock root)   1 ounce
Matricaria recutita (chamomile flower)   1 ounce

If gas and bloating worsen with PMS, enjoy one or more of the following beverage and culinary herbs as part of your daily eating patterns the week before bleeding, or add 1 ounce of any one of the following to your herbal formula to be taken through the month:

Matricaria recutita (chamomile flowers): calming; taste slightly bitter
Zingiber officinale (ginger root): warming; use in small amounts to taste
Achillea millefolium (yarrow flowers): vulnerary bitter tonic; tastes bitter;
    avoid during early pregnancy

If diarrhea occurs with PMS, add:

Rubus villosus (blackberry root)   1 ounce
Matricaria recutita (chamomile flower)   1 ounce

Herbs and Nutrition for PMS Types

Type A (anxiety) treatment includes reducing all fat intake (especially animal fat), decreasing refined sugar intake, and balancing the magnesium-to-calcium ratio. Pyridoxine (B_6) found in whole grains added to the daily diet reduces excess estrogen and increases progesterone levels. Herbs that are nervine relaxants and hepatics are important, such as skullcap *(Scutellaria spp.)* and vervain *(Verbena officinalis)*.

Type C (food cravings) may respond well to evening primrose oil; take 1,000 milligrams daily at least three days before signs and symptoms develop, and until menses. It is helpful to increase intake of vitamin B_6, magnesium (300–600 milligrams), zinc, and manganese. Besides improving blood sugar control, chromium also increases serotonin levels. Herbs that help stabilize blood sugar include the bitters *Taraxacum* (dandelion) and *Achillea* (yarrow).

Cravings may be relieved by herbal nutritive tonics, especially edible seaweeds, nervines, and hepatics; all are incorporated in the formula provided in this chapter. Ensure adequate protein metabolism with herbs that promote hearty digestive function. It only takes a small amount of *Artemisia vulgaris* (mugwort) to improve digestion, but even small amounts should be avoided if a woman with PMS is also trying to get pregnant.

Type H (hyperhydration) may be helped by adding magnesium to the diet (or take supplements for six weeks to see if it helps). Vitamin E and evening primrose oil, taken at least ten days prior to menses, will reduce breast tenderness and swelling. To correct this imbalance decrease use of nicotine, caffeine, sugar, and salt. These steps lessen dependence on herbal formulas that incorporate diuretics such as *Taraxacum* (dandelion leaf), *Petroselinium crispus* (parsley), *Achillea millefolium* (yarrow herb), or the urinary antiseptic, *Arctostaphylos* (uva-ursi leaf). Bitters are also helpful through a complex stimulation of natural processes in the body.

Type P (cramping) can be relieved by decreasing intake of animal protein, substituting more vegetarian-based meals for two weeks prior to menses. Magnesium, calcium, and evening primrose oil may also relieve cramps.

Type S (skin) may be relieved by reducing intake of animal fats and calcium supplements, and emphasizing vegetable proteins and high-calcium foods such as greens. Fruits and complex carbohydrates also help clear skin. Useful herbs include hormonal tonics such as *Vitex* (chasteberry) or *Angelica sinensis* (dong quai root), along with alteratives such as *Rumex crispus* (yellow dock). Diuretics such as fresh parsley in salads or *Taraxacum* (dandelion leaf) assist elimination, while nervine tonics such as *Leonurus* (motherwort herb) address the stress that leads to hormonal acne.

Supplements

Daily recommendations include:

> magnesium: 1,000 milligrams
>
> calcium: 800 milligrams
>
> zinc: 15–50 milligrams
>
> vitamin B_6: 2–50 milligrams
>
> niacin: 15 milligrams
>
> vitamin C: 1–5 grams

Other Points

Herbal treatment must be undertaken in the context of creating sacred space. When you cannot actually leave the world behind, nervine herbs and nutritive tonics help you remain relaxed and centered. If you can't go to the mountain, herbs can bring the mountain refuge to you.

Visualization

You may change the following affirming visualization into your own words. You may have another person read it to you, or you may tape it and play it when you wish to tune in and release tension, making room for fresh energy. If you hear it often during times of stress, soon the words will take on new meaning in your life. If you become familiar with the essence of the words, you will be able to tap into this refuge of the spirit at any time.

Stop what you are doing and breathe. Feel your body. Acknowledge how it feels, not how you wish it to feel. Relax with your next breath. Watch your breath come in. Watch your breath go out. Visualize a pink glow of health in your center, low down in your pelvis. See it in your mind's eye, washing over your womb, with soft, pink, healing light . . . as light as angels of mercy. Even if you have had surgery, even if there is only the body memory of a reproductive system, imagine it intact, healthy, and whole, surrounded by a pale, rosy glow. Let that vision of perfect wholeness heal old wounds now. Be touched, be safe, be at home in your body. Be at home within your larger body: a family of women who gave you life from their bodies. Thank them and perhaps forgive them if any of their actions have caused you any distress. Forgive yourself for choices you have made that you would make differently now. Be at home in a larger body still . . . the celestial body we call earth, rich with flowers and green healing plants for you, her daughter. Breathe deeply. Feel your body. Relax any tension with your next slow breath. Watch your breath come in. Watch your breath go out. Let your attention be brought gently but completely to this place where you sit, the day you are in . . . Open your eyes and know that you have a home. It is safe. You can be whole. Let your highest vision be made real.

5

Dysmenorrhea: Painful or Difficult Menstrual Cycles

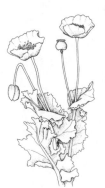

Definition

Dysmenorrhea means a painful or difficult menstrual flow. That includes an irregular menstrual cycle. More commonly, dysmenorrhea describes pain, fatigue, cramps, menstrual blood clots, and heavy bleeding (see also Chapter 6: Menorrhagia and Chapter 9: Fibroids).

If you have dysmenorrhea that is worsened by PMS (premenstrual syndrome), refer to Chapter 4: PMS, too. Fortunately, our time of the month can be made easier by using natural treatments to balance hormones.

Symptoms and Signs

Dysmenorrhea causes pain immediately before menstruation or on the first day of flow. Typically it peaks at the end of the first twenty-four hours of bleeding, but women have every known variation of possible timings for the pain. There is cramping, with digestive symptoms such as bloating, gas, diarrhea, or constipation. Pain comes and goes, and often centers in the lower abdomen. This can spread to the lower back, buttocks, inner thighs, and vulva. Women liken the symptoms to labor pains; it can feel sharp and cause them to gasp. The pain can also be dull and cause fatigue and depression.

Cause

If periods are irregular by a few months, the gaps may be due to one ovary not functioning well in response to hormonal messages. Other causes of painful periods are tension, taut nerves and muscles, excess inflammatory prostaglandins, and a poor level of fitness combined with poor nutritional habits.

Conventional Medical Care

The conventional approach is to use aspirin or other pain-relieving drugs, including narcotics. Prostaglandin inhibitors (including aspirin for mild pain) are also used. Stronger drugs of this type include ibuprofen, Advil, Aleve, Motrin, Naprosyn, or Naproxen. Typically they work for a while, then stop being effective, or ever-larger amounts are required to take the edge off cramping and pain.

When women are saturated with these pain medications it is best to keep taking them while starting herbal treatment, reducing the number of pills gradually, month by month. Herbs cannot mimic these drugs; they work in a different way. Women will experience fewer rebound effects when they let their body set the pace of weaning off these symptom-suppressing agents as their health slowly returns.

Primary dysmenorrhea is seen in orthodox medical circles as occurring without any known cause. It is treated with sex steroids, analgesics, or sedatives for psychogenic factors (originating in the mind). Secondary dysmenorrhea, due to known causes such as endometriosis or fibroids, is treated with drugs prior to surgery.

Herbal Treatment

Integrated medicine for dysmenorrhea is based on the idea that this condition is usually a problem of *function* rather than of organic pathology. Difficult menstrual cycles respond beautifully to herbal treatment for normalizing function. In the case of dysmenorrhea caused by organic disease, herbal therapy can still provide a woman with support if her treatment team wants to use everything possible for her best recovery.

Plants that contain phytosterols (compounds in plants with an effect on human hormone metabolism) balance a woman's hormones over a few months or cycles to trigger her "reset button." She can usually carry on after that point without such herbs, given good nutrition; a woman's own rhythm is usually reestablished in a matter of months.

In other civilizations, cramps are made bearable by the use of pain-diminishing herbs, but the wise women know that this is not a symptom to suppress; this is the way the uterus practices contractions, like exercising any muscle. How else would young women build up strength gradually, a little each month, to handle the heavy contractions of a future birth with relative elasticity?

Herbs used for painful cramps or contractions are not like modern nerve-blocking agents. With the right plant medicine, the relief comes from getting *with* the flow, not jamming it up. Aching back muscles are not a punishment; they remind women how important exercise and good posture are, so that later when they carry a baby on their hip several times a day, their back, legs, and stomach muscles are fit and supple. Places that ache may be rubbed, pains lessened, but a woman's body learns how to cycle with ease.

Because the herbs described in this chapter are both effective and mild when used correctly, most women take herbal treatments for dysmenorrhea in three-month phases until positive results are achieved. It is rare to use a monthly herbal "push" for one to two years, though this has been known to work in extreme cases in which stress and nutrition are not improved.

If taking the herbs as recommended doesn't relieve symptoms in three months, ask for better quality herbs, check the diagnosis, then try another three months before giving up—especially if it is a long-standing condition and there is no immediate health risk. For every year a condition has existed, it may take a solid month of herbal therapy to effect a real improvement that can be maintained after the herbs are stopped.

An alternative is to switch to milder herbs that have similar actions when herbs are used six months or longer, or for long-term maintenance of health (six months to two years). Once symptoms are better it is common to take this herbal mainte-nance regimen of milder herbs (see Chapter 1: Herbal Glossary for mild herbs, listed first for each action). Usually this herbal regimen is followed for the same number of months that the stronger herbal treatment was taken. You switch from stronger to milder herbal treatments when your periods don't hurt anymore.

Herbal treatments commonly fail due to two causes: stopping the treatment too soon, or taking too small a dose (expensive retail extracts taken in drops).

If there are signs of worsening health after two or three months of taking the herbs, double-check the source of the plants and the choice of herbal regimen, re-assess the diagnosis, or try another healing method.

Two Types of Dysmenorrhea

The holistic approach to treating a woman with dysmenorrhea divides types of functional disorder into two broad categories: "congestive" and "spastic." The first category is characterized by pelvic congestion. The second is linked to spasm of the internal organs including painful cramps of the uterus, which is one big muscle. A woman may have elements of both types. Fortunately, the herbs have more than one action; many are found in both formulas for this reason.

Congestive Dysmenorrhea   Congestive dysmenorrhea is associated with poor circulation, excess weight, constipation, fibroids (benign uterine growths), heavy blood loss, and a dull or aching pain. Cramping builds up during the first few days before the menstrual flow. Cramps may diminish fully or partially with the flow because the exit of menstrual blood relieves the congestion. This pelvic congestion is also associated with certain PMS signs: breast swelling, tenderness, general water retention, and irritability. The herbal actions that help are:

- anti-spasmodics such as *Viburnum opulus* (cramp bark)
- mild diuretics that do not over-tax the kidneys, such as *Taraxacum* (dandelion), *Trifolium* (red clover), and *Petroselinum* (parsley)
- digestive tonics, aperients, and hepatics to encourage better liver function and intestinal elimination, such as *Rumex crispus* (yellow dock), *Taraxacum* (dandelion), *Humulus* (hops), and *Verbena officinalis* (vervain)
- hormonal tonics such as *Vitex agnus-castus* (chasteberry) or *Cimicifuga* (black cohosh)
- nervines with an affinity for the reproductive system, such as *Matricaria* (chamomile), *Leonurus* (motherwort), *Verbena officinalis* (vervain) or the stronger *Valeriana* (valerian)
- circulatory tonics, to improve arterial blood flow, such as *Rosmarinus officinalis* (rosemary) or *Zingiber spp.* (ginger root); herbs to improve venous drainage include *Aesculus hippocastunum* (horse chestnut seed), while lymphatic tonics include *Calendula officinalis* (calendula flowers) and *Galium aparnine* (cleavers herb).

Herbal Formula for Congestive Dysmenorrhea

Vitex agnus-castus (vitex, chasteberry seed)	2 ounces
Caulophyllum thalictroides (blue cohosh root)	1 ounce
Achillea millefolium (yarrow flower)	2 ounces
Rumex crispus (yellow dock root)	1 ounce
Leonurus cardiaca (motherwort herb)	1 ounce
Viburnum spp. (black haw or cramp bark)	2 ounces
Zingiber spp. (ginger root)	¼ ounce

Take according to standard directions and dosage (see Chapter 2), whether as tea, tincture, or capsules, throughout the month.

Spastic Dysmenorrhea   Spastic dysmenorrhea is associated with periods in younger women, many of whom have not been pregnant. Pain is due mainly to uterine muscle spasms. There may be fewer PMS symptoms than with congestive dysmenorrhea, but emotional factors play a large role here. The cramps are more severe at the onset of flow. This is a symptom of a background state of excess tension in the nervous system in which blood flow, warmth, and oxygen are cut off from the muscles by the force of menstrual spasms. There is less dull, aching pain than in congestive dysmenorrhea, but there is more sharp pain. In both cases, the pain is due to lack of blood and oxygen in the muscle tissue. This pain may be felt all the way down the legs. Women with spastic dysmenorrhea have a low pain threshold, which is especially noticeable at menses.

Predisposing factors for spastic dysmenorrhea include a high state of tension in the sympathetic nervous system. Messages from the sympathetic nervous system tell our muscles to tighten up and get ready for fight or flight. When women are under chronic stress, the nerve messages to the uterus are already humming with tension. When the uterus goes through its normal monthly cleansing, the uterine muscle must contract hard to slough off the menstrual lining. But the surrounding structures are already as taut as wires. This causes uterine contractions to be painful, although nature designed them to be a rhythmic pulse of a relaxed womb. Nervine relaxants and antispasmodics are in the following formulas for women with cramps of this description.

When sympathetic nervous tension is high in the womb, it may show up elsewhere: nervous diarrhea, irritable bowel syndrome, tension headaches, or nervous bladder tension.

Saying that the emotional factor is significant does not mean painful symptoms are all in a woman's mind. You are one integrated organism, not compartmentalized into physical and emotional bodies. For this reason, physically relaxing herbs as mild as hyssop and chamomile can have a strong effect since they are also calming to emotional states. Another calming herb is pasque flower (not to be confused with passionflower). Pasque flower (*Anemone pulsatilla)* is used to treat inflammatory pain of the reproductive tract of either gender.

Women with spastic dysmenorrhea commonly have high levels of progesterone and a prostaglandin called PGF2-alpha. Such women respond well to phytoestrogenic and relaxing herbs, such as *Trifolium pratense* (red clover), *Humulus lupulus* (hops), and *Angelica sinensis* (dong quai), rather than *Vitex* (chasteberry).

Herbal Formula for Spastic Dysmenorrhea

Cimicifuga racemosa (black cohosh root)	2 ounces
Trifolium pratense (red clover flower)	1 ounce
Viburnum opulus (cramp bark)	2 ounces

SUGGESTED ACTIVITIES FOR BABY

One to Three Months

When changing baby, move arms over head, push knees up like a bicycle exercise, gently push feet when he's on his tummy.

Place him on his tummy and put bright objects in front of him to look at. Take bumper pad away for short periods of time so he can see out.

Move a bright toy in front of him and let him follow it with his eyes.

Show him a favorite toy and have it disappear from his view, then reappear.

Put rattle in baby's hand, put his hand up so he can see it.

Help him put his hands together, and hold them in front of his face to see them.

phrases -- "baby's leg," "baby's hair," "bath," etc.

Place him nearby when family eats; have him in the kitchen when you make the dinner.

Take him for walks, rides, to visit friends.

JB:jh
2/2-1

7/6/87

Valeriana officinalis (valerian root)	1 ounce
Humulus lupulus (hops flower)	1 ounce
Anemone pulsatilla (pasque flower herb)	1 ounce

Follow standard preparation and dosage (see Chapter 2), and drink throughout the menstrual cycle for a minimum of two months; three months or more is better, but after the second month if pain is lessened or if valerian disagrees with you, you may replace the valerian with chamomile. There is so little valerian in this formula that it shouldn't make you feel tired, but it isn't necessary to take it after two menstrual cycles unless tension continues to be a problem. If tension does continue, continue to take the valerian if it helps.

Nine out of ten people are relaxed by valerian, but some experience an occasional paradoxical increase of nervous tension. If you have an adverse reaction to valerian root, please replace it with either:

Matricaria recutita (chamomile flower)	2 ounces
Passiflora incarnata (passionflower herb)	2 ounces

OR

Scutellaria spp. (skullcap herb)	2 ounces

If you have heavy bleeding due to fibroids, add:

Mitchella repens (partridgeberry)	1 ounce

Please see Chapter 6: Menorrhagia or Chapter 9: Fibroids for additional information.

For Pain and Cramps

Valeriana officinalis (valerian) (or passionflower or skullcap herb)	1 ounce
Viburnum opulus (cramp bark)	1 ounce

Use as much of this formula as you need for short-term improvement in the quality of life. The combination of *equal parts* of cramp bark and valerian tea or tincture can be helpful in the early stages of cramping. You may use as little as 15 drops or as much as ½ ounce of tincture in a glass of water every fifteen to thirty minutes. It combines well with a cup of hot cinnamon tea (or tincture in hot water), or with other warming digestive herbs such as ginger and rosemary.

When larger amounts (two doses of ½ ounce tincture) of the valerian/cramp bark combination are ineffective, or when the cramps have progressed to a severe stage, preventive measures and external applications are more effective than bigger, stronger doses of herbal analgesics (anodynes).

If you are taking the herbal formula, and you still need pain killers at high doses every month for more than three months, it is a serious indication that the formula is not able to do the job. Either the formula must be changed or the diagnosis rechecked. Pain-relieving herbs more specific to ovaries, fallopian tubes, or pelvic structures exist (also see Chapter 12: Endometriosis and Chapter 9: Fibroids) but a crystal-clear understanding of the pain's cause is required in order to be effective.

External Herbal Therapies

If stillness appeals instead of exercise, put a small bag of sea salt (one or two pounds; it's heavy) in a heat-resistant container in a 325 degrees F oven for 30 minutes. When the salt is heated, pour it into a cloth that can be folded so that the temperature is pleasant on the abdomen. This can also be placed over the lower back (sacrum) to relieve cramps. The salt can be reheated and reused as often as desired.

Rubbing a few drops or a small palmful of undiluted essential oil of ginger over the abdomen or lower back is both pain-relieving and warming. Essential oils are available at herb shops or natural food stores, or from mail-order companies (see Appendix for Suppliers). Ginger oil is not very expensive, and it smells great. Imagine that you are on vacation in a tropical paradise as you massage it in and feel its sunny, earthy heat seep into your cramped muscles.

Nutrition

Taking evening primrose oil helps reduce pain. This is partly because it nourishes the insulating fatty cell layers surrounding nerve tissue while beneficially affecting specific prostaglandins related to pain and inflammation. Evening primrose oil may also help with the underlying imbalance of hormones, but this is less certain. It does need to be balanced with other essential fatty acids taken as a supplement. The ratio of omega-3 to omega-6 oils can be maintained by taking evening primrose oil and a product of omega-3 oils, such as Max-EPA.

Avoiding animal proteins (eggs, dairy, red meat) ten days before bleeding is helpful, as they increase the levels of prostaglandin, which is implicated in pain. Some women do best to cut out or reduce overall levels of animal products throughout the month; however, cold water fish (salmon, trout) are helpful.

Calcium from plant sources (sesame seeds, almonds, and dark green, leafy vegetables) is also helpful; absorption is aided by vitamins A, C, and D. Carrots help menstrual blood to be more easily passed and make periods less painful. An glass of fresh carrot juice (8 to 10 ounces) each morning, beginning two days to a week before bleeding, is especially recommended for women with clotting.

Eat lightly one day a week for a few months to accelerate decongestion, mainly relying on liquids such as vegetable broths, fruit/vegetable juices, and herb teas. It makes things feel a lot looser—more "freed up" inside.

Supplements

Daily recommendations include:

evening primrose oil: 3,000 milligrams (two 500-milligram capsules three times per day)

omega-3 oils such as Max-EPA: take as directed

vitamin A: 4,000 IU

vitamin B6: 2 milligrams

vitamin C: 1–5 grams

vitamin D: 400 IU

calcium: food sources are best, or try 800 milligrams citrate, chelate, or calcium phosphate

magnesium: 1,000 milligrams

zinc: 15 milligrams

niacin: 15 milligrams

Other Points

Exercise is strongly recommended for relieving any type of difficult or painful period. Especially good are stretching, walking, yoga, Tai Chi, or aerobic activity, for ten to thirty minutes a day throughout the month.

During cramps, women find almost immediate relief by lying flat on their back on a firm surface or floor, knees up to the chest. Rocking gently back and forth relieves pressure and gets blood through the pelvis, bringing oxygen and other benefits along with warming the muscles.

Another way to encourage elimination in dysmenorrhea is to squat or crouch down with your hands on the floor, like a frog settling down in a nice, sun-warmed mud puddle. It helps if you are in a warm place. Find your center so that you know how far to go without losing your balance, then rock back and forth. Feel the resistance and pressure in your lower back and abdomen melt away.

Orgasms provide complete and immediate relief of tension and pain. You do not have to have penetration to have an orgasm, but there is no reason to avoid gentle intercourse during bleeding if it brings pleasure and release.

6

Menorrhagia and Hypermenorrhea: Heavy Menstrual Bleeding

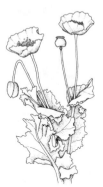

Definition

Menorrhagia means excessive menstrual flow. A similar term, used less frequently these days, is *hypermenorrhea.* Hypermenorrhea refers to blood loss in normal amounts, but continued for too long—eight or more days each cycle. Menorrhagia can mean gushing rivers or big clots lost during a normal length of bleeding time; it may even mean that most of the blood loss happens quickly in extreme floods during the first day or two.

These terms are both different than *metrorrhagia*, which means bleeding from the womb *between* normal menses—a potentially more serious symptom.

Dysfunctional Uterine Bleeding (DUB) is a term for abnormal shedding of the uterine lining when no obvious reason can be found.

Symptoms and Signs

What qualifies as "excessive" menstrual blood loss? Like the "normal" length of a menstrual cycle, the definition depends more on an increase from what has been healthy and normal for a particular woman than on any defined amount. The typical pattern of healthy bleeding is to start slowly, lose a lot of blood by the end of the first or second day, then taper off in three to six days. If a woman soaks through more than one tampon or pad per hour for more than three hours in a row, she needs to take a rest to prevent heavier blood loss. If there is a mixed pattern, with rapid and heavy bleeding that slows down for a few hours between "flooding" episodes, it still requires care. Comparing each cycle to previous menses is helpful, as is recording any special stresses or other causes of an unusually heavy period.

The most common symptom of DUB is spotting or bleeding between periods. There may also be heavy periods lasting longer than eight days, or frequent periods with short cycles (bleeding every eighteen to twenty-one days). Symptoms of DUB may improve or worsen at unpredictable times. Excess bleeding of any pattern may lead to anemia, so fatigue and weakness are other signs to watch for (see Chapter 7: Anemia).

Cause

In the case of uncomplicated menorrhagia, the body is getting rid of a great deal of menstrual material. Usually this is because of some temporary abnormality in the uterus. This might not be a serious health abnormality. For instance, missing an ovulation happens more frequently than many menstruating women realize.

Common causes of heavy bleeding include fibroids, endometrial polyps, and overgrowth of the uterine lining, sometimes due to lack of ovulation. Other causes include inappropriate diet (especially malnutrition), vitamin K deficiency, excess salt in the diet, red meat, caffeine, excess aspirin, or a calcium deficiency. This last condition is not best treated by taking in more calcium, since the deficiency is often one of absorption, availability, balance, and excretion.

Hormonal causes for heavy bleeding may be separate from nutritional causes, but it is common for an inappropriate diet to aggravate a hormone imbalance. Commercial dairy products and other animal foods lead to endocrine imbalance. A simple diet based on grains, vegetables, fruit, and plant proteins will benefit women in many ways.

Low thyroid is one of the endocrine conditions known to result in heavy menstrual blood loss. So is adrenal or pituitary dysfunction. It is possible to get an infection severe enough to make the uterus jettison a thick uterine lining, but this usually clears up when the infection is treated adequately. Drugs, including anticoagulants (i.e., aspirin), corticosteroid anti-inflammatories, and digitalis may trigger frequent periods, whether or not each period is heavy.

Another cause of heavy periods may be fragile blood vessels and circulation problems—usually poor blood flow to and from the pelvis.

A deep emotional shock can also jolt the hormones, nervous system, and uterus into a heavy blood loss; this can also cause metrorrhagia.

In holistic therapies, regular heavy periods are seen as a sign of vascular congestion. Local obstructions are the most common cause (see "Congestive Dysmenorrhea" in Chapter 5). Benign fibroids or uterine polyps may prevent uterine blood from leaving the vagina. Even missing an ovulation can result in a thicker uterine lining that month, and a heavier bleed. If this happens regularly, the various reasons for skipping ovulations must be sorted out to understand the underlying cause.

Other causes of heavy bleeding with each period are inflammation with or without infections, such as endometriosis, endometritis (inflammation of the uterine lining itself), pelvic inflammatory disease (PID), salpingitis (inflamed or infected fallopian tubes), or possibly tumors.

During menopause, a decrease in estrogen levels makes the vagina more susceptible to friction and bleeding, yet an excess of estrogen at any age can cause a tendency to bleed. Bleeding other than during normal menses can also be a complication of pregnancy or even a symptom of cancer.

If a woman has DUB, it usually means that she has excess estrogen, causing an imbalance in the hormones that stimulate the endometrium (uterine lining) each menstrual cycle. Excess estrogen can result from being overweight, drinking coffee and colas, polycystic ovary disease, or problems in younger women with hormones of the hypothalamus, pituitary, or ovary. Women in their late thirties and early forties who do not ovulate may also develop high levels of estrogen since they are not producing post-ovulation progesterone to balance estrogen. In all these cases, the uterine lining usually looks normal unless it shows long-term changes, as when there is excess estrogen, the diseases excess estrogen may cause, or cancer.

Women from Love Canal to the Rio Grande have many opportunities for developing any one of these conditions. Our Western culture's sedentary lifestyle and poor food choices, mixed in with a heavy dose of exposure to environmental toxins, is thought to be partly responsible for numerous reproductive disorders. However, heavy bleeding is more commonly a reflection of a change in uterine function, rather than a life-threatening problem.

Conventional Medical Care

The conventional medical view is that if any recognizable growths, infections, or inflammation are present, the abnormal bleeding is more serious than a simple imbalance leading to dysfunction. Some herbalists view these more obvious signs as outgrowths of the same dysfunction that caused the symptom of heavy periods. Abnormal uterine bleeding with no organic lesions or recognizable cause is the reason for almost one-fourth of all gynecological surgeries. Herbalists feel that there are too many surgeries performed, and prefer to treat a functional imbalance more conservatively if dangerous causes have been ruled out.

Heavy bleeding is usually painless, though a woman may feel pressure or aching. The symptom of pain with abnormal bleeding always requires a call to a licensed care provider to rule out problems.

The conventional treatment for irregular menses characterized by heavy blood loss without other disease is conservative. Often a doctor will recommend treating any anemia, but the heavy bleeding may require no treatment. Drugs to induce ovulation are used for a thickened endometrial lining due to anovulation. A D&C (dilation and curettage) is frequently used for polyps or heavy bleeding of unknown origin. However, this and other forms of reducing a thickened lining, such as burning (cauterization) or freezing (cryosurgery), only treats the symptom on the assumption that the body will right itself in a few cycles. More invasive disease may necessitate a hysterectomy.

If menorrhagia (heavy or prolonged bleeding) accompanies the separate symptom of metrorrhagia (bleeding between periods), a woman may still be able to use natural approaches, but the wisest course is to get a diagnosis first.

Conventional treatment for DUB, depending on a woman's age, is the birth control pill, which combines high doses of estrogen and progesterone. When women past menopause have vaginal bleeding, it is best to see a licensed care provider.

Herbal Treatment

The appropriate herbs for treating metrorrhagia depend on the cause. For spotting without a more serious disease, the following astringent, tonic Herbal Formula I, will provide the body with the opportunity to heal. For cervical erosion, see Chapter 11: Cervical Dysplasia. For polyps see Chapter 9: Fibroids, since the approach to these two types of benign uterine growth share herbal actions. For complications of pregnancy, please see Part 4: "Healthy Reproduction." Cancers of the reproductive tract may also be a cause of bleeding between cycles. This topic requires more space than this book allows; please see *Breast Cancer* by Steve Austin, N.D., and Cathy Hitchcock, and *Women's Bodies, Women's Wisdom,* by Christiane Northrup, M.D. (see Bibliography).

Since DUB has so many causes, there can be more than one herbal approach. The holistic objective is to reestablish a longer cycle, promote natural ovulation, support the corpus luteum in producing sufficient progesterone after ovulation, and prevent problems of self-repair associated with anemia and reduce unopposed estrogen.

It isn't enough to state that the cause of heavy bleeding is hormone imbalance, a fibroid, or a chronic infection. Where did the fibroid get its signal to overgrow? If environment and nutrition are not improved, one condition or another will probably develop from a background state of poor health. Heavy bleeding due to a chronic infection may clear up with antimicrobial herbs, but we are exposed to infections frequently; why did this infection take hold? If menorrhagia is due to hormone imbalance, perhaps causing an obstruction such as a fibroid, the "cure" is the wellness of the woman—not simply removal of fibroids. The herbs I list in this chapter will help achieve that state of wellness.

Once the cause of heavy menstrual bleeding is determined, the aim of herbal treatment is to improve circulation, using astringent herbs to reduce tissue overgrowth (benign uterine fibroids are common) and to tone and tighten the endometrial lining to its optimal thickness for different phases of the month. Formulas combine herbs for balancing estrogen and progesterone with herbs to support the whole orchestra of hormonal voices. This includes attention to the thyroid, adrenal glands, and pancreas.

The following Herbal Formula I includes herbal tonics for hormone balance and circulatory stimulants to normalize blood supply to tissue. In combination, these herbs affect levels of oxygen and glucose, which in turn affect energy levels. Herbs that add minerals have a nutritive role in addition to antimicrobials that help support a woman's immune defenses so they can neutralize abnormal cells on their own. The uterine astringent tonics, such as *Anemone pulsatilla* (pasque flower), fresh *Capsella bursa-pastoris* (shepherd's purse), or *Mitchella repens* (partridgeberry), combine far-reaching herbal actions to shrink benign growths, including fibroids.

The holistic herbal treatment of menorrhagia extends beyond clearing the symptom to reversing the underlying causes. The immediate goal of normalizing blood flow may include taking care of any anemia, whether obvious or borderline. Prevention is important to protect women with chronic heavy periods from vulnerability to further illness due to weakness.

Heavy bleeding that does not respond to herbal care for balancing natural function within three periods must be referred to a practitioner. In severe cases, or with frequent spotting between cycles, a diagnosis is advised within two weeks. These symptoms may mean nothing, or they may be the tip of a more serious iceberg, especially as we grow older. No matter what the symptom, there is no need for panic. As long as you are breathing you are a candidate for holistic herbal treatment, whether or not it is combined with conventional care.

Herbal Formula I is for treating menorrhagia, and it has several possible variations.

Herbal Formula I

Caulophyllum thalictroides (blue cohosh root)	2 ounces
Vinca major (periwinkle herb)	2 ounces
Urtica dioica (nettles)	3 ounces
Mitchella repens (partridgeberry or squaw vine herb)	6 ounces
Berberis aquifolium (Oregon grape root bark)	3 ounces

Calendula officinalis (calendula flower)	2 ounces
Glycyrrhiza officinalis (licorice root)	2 ounces
Rosmarinus officinalis (rosemary leaf)	5 ounces

This is best made as a combination of extracts. Though the standard infusion is one ounce of herb mixture per pint (two cups) of water, this works better in three cups of water. Even so, it tastes bitter. The licorice makes the other herbs with intense flavors easier on the digestion.

If you prefer to make tea, for lower cost or to avoid alcohol, add flavor herbs to taste. Start by increasing the quantity of licorice root to 4 ounces unless you cannot use licorice root due to problems with water retention. Substitute to taste with basil leaf and your favorite flavor of herb (orange peel, lemon verbena herb, hibiscus flower, fennel seed). Women who have taken this combination say that they grow to love it after a while. Even though there are roots mixed with leaves, this formula can be steeped: 1 ounce of herb mixture to three cups of water, fifteen to twenty minutes, covered. Strain and drink one cup three times a day, or two large cups twice a day.

Alternatively, you can make ground herbs into capsules. Take two #00 capsules with a glass of water and food two to four times a day.

Whatever form you choose, continue taking this formula for a minimum of three months.

If your symptoms are responding slowly yet your general health is good, you may continue taking the formula for six or more months. You have time to continue this gentle way of getting to the underlying cause unless worsening health signs indicate you need to check with your health care provider. For such long-term rebuilding of your reproductive balance, skip the herbs one day per week to allow your body to rest. If you have questions, continue checking in with a health care provider who understands your health goals. Most physicians are not taught about herbs and so may feel suspicious about your use of them. Herbalists in your area or national organizations listed in the Resources may be able to provide you with information that will be specific to you.

When you reach menopause, fibroids, polyps, endometriosis, and other non-malignant uterine causes of menorrhagia will diminish with the drop in estrogen. Hang on and keep taking the formula if you can until then. As long as you are not endangering your health (get second opinions), you have all the time in the world.

For quick relief from heavy bleeding, take as a separate extract: one teaspoon of tincture of <u>fresh</u> *Capsella bursa-pastoris* (shepherd's purse herb), diluted in one three-ounce glass of water every hour until bleeding slows or stops.

For chronic heavy bleeding, this dose may be taken twice a day, morning and evening, for a minimum of three months. If it tastes too bitter for your taste buds, you can stir a little honey into each teaspoon dose.

With ovulation pain (sometimes called by its Germanic medical name, *mittelschmerz*), add:

Viburnum opulus (cramp bark)	3 ounces
Cimicifuga racemosa (black cohosh)	3 ounces

These are also useful additions for excessive cramping and pain with heavy bleeding due to clots.

When there is heavy bleeding with clotting, Herbal Formula I will help. However, there are herbs that are more specific for clotting. In health, our enzymes have time to break menstrual clumps and clots down to a runny liquid. And when blood clots are small, we don't notice them. The real problem with menstrual blood clots is that they are too big to exit through the small os (the cervical opening from the uterus to the vagina). Larger clots signify an imbalance in hormones, diet, or stress. Too rapid a sloughing off of the uterine lining will also cause clots. Try the following formula for clotting:

Herbal Formula II

Vitex agnus-castus (chasteberry)	4 ounces
Rumex crispus (yellow dock root)	3 ounces
Foeniculum vulgare (fennel seed)	3 ounces
Mitchella repens (partridgeberry herb)	2 ounces
Rubus idaeus (raspberry leaf)	2 ounces
Urtica dioica (nettle leaf)	2 ounces

Take as a tea: 1 ounce infused for fifteen to twenty minutes in 2 pints (4 cups) of water; take one cup four times a day for two weeks, then one cup three times a day for four weeks, then one cup twice a day for six weeks. Alternatively, you may take this as a combination of extracts: one teaspoon three times a day for three months.

If you have problems with clotting, take a vacation from whatever may be causing you stress. If you can't get away for long, a hot lavender bath and a good cry in the dark don't require more than a little time away from the usual cares of the day.

Nutrition

To relieve blood clotting, add fresh carrot juice to your diet ten days before and during your period. At least just before and during the period drop dairy products and meat. You may leave them out of the diet altogether for a few months (three) for the best results.

In general, enjoy moderate amounts of high-quality protein (lean fish, beans, and grains) along with mineral-rich foods such as green leafy vegetables. If you need high amounts of protein to match your physical needs, choose fresh fish and sea foods.

Include seaweeds such as dulse and kelp to aid metabolism. Eat high-fiber foods, and cut down on caffeine intake. Avoid pleasure drugs and excess aspirin intake.

Supplements

Daily recommendations include:

vitamin K: 45–65 milligrams

vitamin C: 200 milligrams, or up to 5 grams with bioflavonoids and
   extra rutin

vitamin E: 200–800 IU

Liquid Iron Formula for building blood (see Chapter 7: Anemia) or food-
   based supplements such as the formula in Chapter 7 if chronic heavy
   bleeding leads to anemia

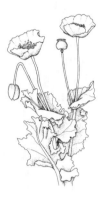

7

*Iron-Deficiency
Anemia*

Definition

The term "anemia" is not really a diagnosis; it is a sign of several possible imbalances. Even mild anemia is a sign women should not ignore. Taking iron supplements only treats the symptom.

The first problem with having blood that is low in iron isn't just an iron problem; it's the lack of oxygen to tissue and cells which this iron deficiency causes.

In health, iron and our red blood cells do a wonderful ballet together to pick up oxygen in the lungs. The iron carries the precious oxygen in its little iron arms all over the body until a waiting cell with open arms receives the oxygen, sending the red blood cell with its empty iron arms back to the lungs for more oxygen. It is a very elegant biochemical performance.

When there isn't enough oxygen, the heart gets the message to pump the red blood cells harder. The red blood cells dance more frenetically to get their few oxygen molecules delivered to the waiting cells. Then the lungs have to work harder, too. First one breathes more deeply, then after a while there is shallow breathing—not a good sign.

Symptoms and Signs

Severe anemia is associated with fatigue (no oxygen-rich "juice" to the muscles), lack of concentration, headaches (not enough oxygen to the brain), irritability, and

66

worse. Amenorrhea (lack of periods), a drop in sex drive, and digestive system symptoms such as jaundice or enlarged spleen may develop.

Extreme anemia can lead to shock if there isn't enough blood volume or blood pressure in the veins and arteries to keep one upright and functioning. There can even be heart failure.

Anemia can creep up gradually with no obvious symptoms, unless one is paying attention to other signals (heavy bleeding, fatigue that can't be explained, feeling cold and tired, looking pale).

The body gives us lots of chances to correct a worsening imbalance. Tissue signs that may be seen include pale skin, fatigue, difficulty breathing, craving for minerals such as magnesium, and a bright red-magenta tongue with a shiny, swollen look, also associated with a vitamin-B$_2$ deficiency. In severe anemia, fingernails may grow oddly, with depressions in the nail bed giving a "spoon" shape. Of course, fatigue and fainting are signs of extreme anemia that may be seen at any time.

Cause

There are many causes of anemia. Iron deficiency is the most common. A common cause of iron-deficiency anemia for women is heavy menstrual bleeding, especially due to uterine fibroids (see Chapter 9). Other kinds of blood loss, such as slow or intermittent bleeding ulcers, any hemorrhage, or traumatic accidents can also bring on iron-deficient anemia. A simple blood test determines the type and cause.

A second cause of anemia is difficulty in making good red blood cells. This is a common result of poor nutrition, in which a low level of usable iron or protein means that fewer healthy red blood cells can be made. Adolescent girls are so busy growing and beginning to menstruate that they may use and lose iron faster than their diet can replace it. Contrary to the old notion that men need the lion's share of protein for physical labor, women need the best protein for a healthy reproductive system. In particular, pregnant women are vulnerable to iron-deficiency anemia because of the high metabolic demands on their red-blood-cell production. Conventional iron supplements may constipate a woman who, if pregnant, is already vulnerable to hemorrhoids and all the problems of a full, heavy pelvic basin. The key here is high-quality protein and complete metabolism, not just bigger amounts of protein (see "Nutrition" later in this chapter).

Other types of anemia not covered here include: a lack of vitamin B$_{12}$, folic acid, vitamin C, and copper, or problems in metabolizing these nutrients, causes larger and less efficient red blood cells to be made.

Fibroids (benign uterine growths; see Chapter 9) are an extremely common cause of iron-deficient anemia and heavy periods because they stimulate heavy blood loss (see "Menorrhagia," Chapter 6).

It may take much longer than two menstrual cycles for the herbs to change the underlying causes of the anemia. If there is no crisis, and especially if there might be some signs of improvement, it is still worthwhile to continue herbal therapy, while adopting a cautious attitude in concert with a trusted health care practitioner.

Another common reason for decreased production of red blood cells is suppression of the bone marrow, as occurs in cancer therapy or radiation for thyroid disorders. Some kidney diseases, or other diseases affecting the spleen, may also cause anemia.

Lastly, poor iron absorption happens after operations to remove portions of the digestive tract. The recommended herbs below cannot hurt, and usually help.

Conventional Medical Care

The conventional treatment is to diagnose the reason for anemia first if it is iron-deficiency anemia, then give iron, often with vitamin C to aid absorption. In extreme cases, iron may have to be given by injection or intravenously.

If a woman takes iron supplements for anemia and doesn't improve within a set time period, it may be assumed that she has a dreadful disease requiring investigation and treatment. In fact, it's possible that all she needs is an ability to assimilate the hard little iron pill better. Supportive ideas now incorporated into standard care include small frequent meals for fatigue, easily digested foods (less spice), and pacing daily activity to avoid breathlessness or dizziness.

Herbal Treatment

In emergencies, the first priority is to stop the blood loss and replace blood volume at the nearest emergency center. After stabilizing such cases, the most holistic treatment is still to work on stopping the bleeding or its recurrence by using astringent herbs, which have a specificity for the body system affected (see "Astringents" in Chapter 1). The Liquid Iron Formula (later in this section) incorporates such astringent herbs.

Mineral-rich plants and nourishing foods often work better than drugstore iron tablets to increase blood volume. Herbs do not rebuild dangerously low red-blood-cell counts as quickly as conventional iron given intravenously or by injection. However, for non-crisis situations, herbs can help rebuild a woman's other functions, rather than simply replacing lost iron. Herbs also are easily digested and do not constipate the person taking them.

Malabsorption of iron is a problem for people who have poor digestive function. Bitter herbs can stir sluggish digestion (see "Bitters" in Chapter 1). We need good production of stomach acid to absorb iron, so excessive use of over-the-counter antacids as a calcium supplement is not the answer (malabsorption is only one of the long-term risks of overuse of antacids; see the Osteoporosis section of Chapter 23: Menopause).

The subject of anemias associated with disease and pathological malabsorption is larger than can be covered here, so if bitter herbs and the Liquid Iron Formula that follows have not significantly improved your healthy red blood cell count in the time indicated below, you should seek answers from your health care provider.

The Liquid Iron Formula that follows provides some iron, as well as other minerals that aid assimilation of iron from foods listed in the "Nutrition" section.

Liquid Iron Formula ("Maid of Iron")

Taraxacum officinale radix (dandelion root)	2 ounces
Taraxacum officinale folia (dandelion leaves)	2 ounces
Urtica dioica (nettle leaf)	2 ounces
Rumex crispus (yellow dock leaves/root)	2 ounces
Berberis vulgaris (barberry root bark)	1 ounce
Prunus armeniaca (dried unsulfured apricots)	4 ounces
Glycyrrhiza glabra (licorice root) (optional)	2 ounces

For flavor, other optional ingredients are (¼ ounce each of any or all):

ginger root

fennel seed

dried orange peel

dried cherries

Cut the fruit into small pieces for maximum absorption. Pour 4 cups of boiling water over 2 ounces of the Liquid Iron Formula mixture. Cover with a good lid so that aromas stay in the brew. Steep for twenty minutes, then strain, pressing out the darker brew from the fruit/plant mixture using a large wooden or non-aluminum utensil (don't use your fingers; you could burn them). If you wish, stir in one to two tablespoons of organic honey or blackstrap molasses to every pint while the herbal liquid is still warm. Keep refrigerated and use up in six months. In a non-emergency situation, take 1 to 3 tablespoons every day (2 to 3 tablespoons during menses), between meals, for a minimum of twenty days before retesting blood counts. Seven days to two months are required to restore iron levels in the blood, as long as no continuous bleeding or other debilitating disease is present. Continue taking this supplement for three months. After that, you may take it regularly or occasionally, as needed.

Leave licorice out of the formula if you dislike its flavor or if you have high blood pressure, water retention, or kidney disease.

If heavy menstrual bleeding is the cause of anemia, add 3 ounces of *one* of the following to the maid of iron formula:

Vinca major (periwinkle herb)
Hamamelis virginiana (witch hazel bark)
Mitchella repens (partridgeberry herb)

If you tend to bleed heavily and haven't got time to make the "Maid of Iron" formula (unexpected heavy bleeding does not always happen conveniently), have fresh plant tincture of shepherd's purse on hand. Use one teaspoon every thirty minutes until bleeding slows or stops. Shepherd's purse can only be depended upon to slow excessive reproductive bleeding when the fresh plant is picked in the right season and immediately made into a tincture (see "Resources" for companies that make it). Glycerin tinctures make shepherd's purse more palatable than alcohol, though both are effective if done well.

It may take much longer than two menstrual cycles for the herbs to change the underlying causes of the anemia. If there is no crisis, and especially if there might be some signs of improvement, it is still worthwhile to continue herbal therapy, while adopting a cautious attitude in concert with a trusted health care practitioner.

If anemia and heavy menstrual bleeding do not respond to the consistent use of the herbs in less than two menstrual cycles, it is important to get a diagnosis. None of the herbal approaches are meant to replace emergency care, but they will support healing.

Nutrition

An alternative to iron supplements is food-source liquid iron, available in natural food stores.

Increase your intake of dark green leafy vegetables, both raw and steamed. Don't overcook vegetables.

If you are anemic and not a vegetarian, consider eating meats, especially liver, temporarily. Buy organic meat when possible. If that is not realistic where you live, skip it. There are other great ways to increase your iron without eating animals or taking store-bought iron pills, which cause constipation.

Increase your intake of vegetables and fruits high in vitamin C: baked potatoes, sweet red and cayenne peppers, broccoli, peaches, citrus, currants.

Take one tablespoon of blackstrap molasses per day, or take a food-source vitamin-B-complex supplement or brewer's yeast.

8
Menstrual Migraines

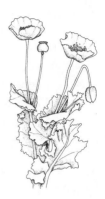

Definition

Menstrual migraines are associated with periods, but they may occur at other times of the month as well. A flood of inflammatory substances into the bloodstream triggers migraines; in menstrual migraines this is complicated by an apparent excess of progesterone before periods.

Migraines are considered to be a problem of the cardiovascular system because they involve blood vessels that expand or contract due to triggers that other people's blood vessels handle more easily. Migraines can be triggered by stress, hormonal changes, or certain foods.

Menstrual migraines can begin as early as puberty and rarely persist past menopause; women usually "outgrow" them by their late thirties.

Symptoms and Signs

A classic sign of migraines is throbbing pain, usually starting and staying on one side of the head, though it may spread to both sides. This is different from regular headaches, however bad they may be, which feel more like a band of tension around the back of the head at the neck or at the temples.

Migraine pain is often localized behind the eye(s). Warning signs include vision changes, seeing a halo around people or objects, a tingling sensation, or altered perceptions and strange moods. There may be colic (intestinal spasm from gas), nausea, and even vomiting. There is usually some abdominal discomfort, along with facial pallor.

71

Migraines typically happen in the morning on weekends and holidays, and peak within four to twenty-four hours, though they fade gradually.

Cluster migraines may happen one to three times a day every few months, and there is usually no warning sign other than the eyes tearing, a stuffy nose, or feelings of agitation. They can be triggered by sensitivity to light and may last from one to forty-eight hours. Pain is often described as "like an ice pick in the eye."

Menstrual migraines usually occur with some form of PMS. They may be the only symptom of PMS, but their treatment is different than other PMS treatments because migraines are both a cardiovascular instability and a state of hormonal imbalance. Please see Chapter 4: PMS to compare suggestions and get additional ideas about nutrition and prevention of the cofactors behind menstrual migraines.

Cause

Menstrual migraines are associated with certain trigger foods such as alcohol (especially red wine), cheese, chocolate, and other foods that contain tyramine, since this amino acid causes the increased release of serotonin. Migraines can also be triggered or aggravated by some medications, including the birth control pill.

Family history plays an important role; fifty percent of people who get migraines have another family member who gets them. Many women who get migraines had childhood colic, periodic abdominal pains, and dizziness as their first indication of what would eventually become a pattern of migraines.

The physical cause is easy to understand: first, blood vessels in the head contract (vasoconstriction), then the body overcompensates and dilates the blood vessels too much. It is the dilation that causes the pain and other symptoms. Not all migraines follow this pattern of vasoconstriction, then dilation, of blood vessels. Though migraines are well-studied, there are some exceptions to every rule. In any case, the herbs work on more than blood vessel tone, so they may help women with atypical migraines. But why do the blood vessels constrict and expand so much in the first place? Menstrual migraines are caused by several cofactors, hormones being the strongest triggers.

Migraines may start with an increase in serotonin—a hormone produced in the brain and from blood platelets—which causes vasoconstriction and triggers platelets to release even more serotonin. In people who don't get migraines, it seems that blood platelets contain the same amount of serotonin, but stimulation by serotonin causes less serotonin release. A simple self-test involves taking caffeine; if it helps prevent or reduce menstrual migraines, then the main herb to use is *Vinca major* (periwinkle herb).

Conventional Medical Care

Aspirin or codeine is given for migraines while they are occurring. In severe attacks, stronger pain relievers may be given in addition to derivatives of ergot (a fungus found on rye). Ergot helps constrict overexpanded blood vessels if taken two hours or more after the onset of a migraine. It can also be given as a suppository. Caffeine also helps, since caffeine constricts blood vessels, but daily use of caffeine (coffee, tea, some diet colas) worsens vascular stability and so worsens menstrual migraines.

Hormone therapy, especially progesterone therapy, is an option because menstrual migraines are triggered by hormone levels that have gotten out of balance.

Daily use of the drug Methysergide may prevent attacks, but it causes side effects and should not be used for more than three months. Methysergide is unsafe during pregnancy.

Other treatments include propranolol, a beta adrenergic blocker used in heart conditions and other disorders.

Herbal Treatment

Herbal actions to relieve migraines include vascular tonics, hepatic alteratives, nervine relaxants, analgesics, and antispasmodics, in addition to hormone-normalizing herbs.

Taraxacum officinale (dandelion root and leaf) is an excellent liver tonic that also reduces water retention premenstrually. A stronger hepatic for this condition is *Verbena officinalis* (vervain herb).

Cimicifuga racemosa (black cohosh root) has hormonal properties, antispasmodic effects, and nervine relaxing properties.

Chrysanthemum parthenium (feverfew) is a *specific* preventative (used to relieve the condition) for all types of migraine, and has been used with menstrual migraines. Fresh feverfew extract or plant daily helps as many as 70% of migraine sufferers. It is a warming bitter—an unusual combination of herbal effects. Most bitters help blood circulate to the digestive system, cooling the body. Feverfew is observed by herbalists to improve digestion and liver function, and to warm a person by opening up peripheral circulation. It is especially good for decreasing severity and frequency of migraine attacks in people with poor digestion and poor circulation to fingers, toes, and the surface of the body.

Tilia spp. (linden blossom) is a traditional migraine remedy. Its demulcent mucilage seems to soothe digestive upsets, as the herb relaxes background muscular tension and helps stabilize or relax inflamed or constricted blood vessels.

Viola odorata (sweet violet) is another demulcent, anti-inflammatory herb with alterative, cooling properties that has been used for some people with migraines. Its properties of soothing digestion and improving elimination (it is a mild diuretic) may also work well with other herbs in combination.

Zingiber spp. (ginger) seems to help with the motion sickness and nausea that worsen migraines. It is a peripheral and central circulatory stimulant, carminative, and caffeine-free metabolic stimulant that affects digestion. Migraines often cause nausea, even vomiting; this herb helps settle the stomach.

Capsicum frutescens (cayenne and other capsicum species of red pepper) depletes Substance P (possibly related to menstrual migraines) in sensory nerves, inhibits platelet aggregation, and is pain-mediating.

Valeriana officinalis (valerian) is both a smooth-muscle anti-spasmodic and a pain reliever via sedation.

Lavender essential oil (*Lavandula spp.*) may be massaged into the temples and forehead (or the entire head and scalp) as often as needed before or during a migraine, along with warm (not hot) essential-oil baths. Heat expands blood vessels, and the goal is to stabilize their sensitivity to change, rather than to expand or contract blood vessels.

Recent aromatherapy studies showed people with headaches also respond well to eucalyptus, peppermint, and rosemary essential oils. Choose the plant oil or combination of these that appeals to your sense of smell.

Herbal Formula

Vinca major (periwinkle herb)	3 ounces
Cimicifuga racemosa (black cohosh root)	3 ounces
Chrysanthemum parthenium (feverfew fresh herb)	3 ounces
Tilia spp. (linden blossom)	2 ounces
Taraxacum officinale (dandelion root)	2 ounces
Taraxacum officinale (dandelion leaf)	1 ounce
Scutellaria lateriflora (skullcap herb)	2 ounces

Because fresh feverfew is usually found as an extract, this formula works well as a tincture combination. The dose is one teaspoon diluted in a glass of water three times a day, taken before meals (up to half an hour before). Taking it before meals aids absorption, but if you forget, take it after meals or without food rather than skipping it entirely. Take the herb mixture each day of the month, but especially from ovulation until bleeding. These herbs work to reduce menstrual migraines, but they are not designed to suppress symptoms once a migraine has begun. They need to be taken consistently for four to ten months before slowly reducing the dose to twice a day, then once a day, to keep menstrual migraines from returning.

Alternatively, many of these herbs make a delicious tea. You can take fresh feverfew and black cohosh as extracts (1 teaspoon each in water, twice a day) in addition to the following tea:

Herbal Tea Formula

Tilia spp. (linden blossom)	2 ounces
Taraxacum officinale (dandelion root)	2 ounces
Taraxacum officinale (dandelion leaf)	1 ounce
Scutellaria lateriflora (skullcap herb)	1 ounce
Viola odorata (sweet violet flower, leaf)	2 ounces

Steep 1 ounce of the herb mixture in 3 cups of water that has just come to the boil; cover and steep for fifteen minutes. Strain and drink one large mug or glass twice a day. Make enough for three days and store in the refrigerator; drink hot or cold, but avoid extreme temperatures since room-temperature liquid is less irritating to nerves. A little honey or lemon may be added to taste.

To take the edge off extreme pain, though it will not stop a migraine, it helps to have a separate bottle of *Valeriana* (valerian root) with or without an equal amount of *Viburnum opulus* (cramp bark). Take 1 to 4 teaspoons of the extract(s) in a little water before the worst symptoms begin. The herbal sister of cramp bark is *Viburnum prunifolium* (black haw), but this will not work as well in menstrual migraines because *V. prunifolium* helps spasms of the uterus and reproductive organs, while cramp bark relaxes spasms in smooth muscle such as the linings of blood vessels.

Case Study: Fresh Feverfew

What about women whose menstrual migraines are aggravated by even a small amount of alcohol? Is there a way around using fresh feverfew tinctures or extracts? Yes, feverfew can be taken in other forms than alcohol extracts, though in my experience dried feverfew has very little power in treating headaches or migraines. In my practice, half the women who have tried feverfew capsules found that they either did not work, or didn't work for very long.

Gwendolyn came to see me three years ago for her unstoppable menstrual migraines. I asked her to keep a feverfew plant growing in a pot. She ate a leaf every day. Some people get small mouth blisters from the bitter-tasting compounds; it helps to disguise the leaf with lettuce in a sandwich or roll it into a ball and swallow it with a glass of water.

Gwen went one step farther: I had her fill a clean one-pint mason jar with fresh, coarsely chopped feverfew, packed evenly but not too tightly, then pour organic apple cider into the jar to an inch above the herb. She put a tight lid on the jar, kept it in a cupboard out of direct light or heat, and shook the contents every day for two weeks. She then strained the herb vinegar out into a clean dark bottle, and took 2 teaspoons a day on salad or in water. She came to love the intensely bitter, invigorating flavor. In seven or eight months, it was the only herbal maintenance she needed.

After a year or so, she reduced her dose to one-half to one teaspoon, according to how she felt. Within two years, she stopped taking the vinegar. Her menstrual migraines only return occasionally when pressures at work build up, and a few months of taking her feverfew vinegar daily resolves the problem. Meanwhile, she has a cheerful abundance of tiny white and yellow chrysanthemum flowers blossoming around her house.

Nutrition

Increase your intake of fresh fruits and vegetables, and incorporate small amounts of warming spices in foods, to taste, three times a week. Choices include cinnamon in apple sauce, a dash of red pepper (cayenne) in salad dressings or other dishes, ginger with vegetables, and curried vegetables.

Avoid chocolate, cheese, alcohol (especially red wine), red grape products, nitrates, MSG (monosodium glutamate), cured meats, caffeine, tobacco, and oranges.

Minimize sugar intake, especially vanilla ice cream.

Quercetin is a flavonoid that improves cardiovascular stability. Though you can take supplements, eating green vegetables, fruit in season, legumes, and whole grains on a regular basis is the best way to get your quercetin.

Supplements

Daily recommendations include:

> vitamin B_2 (niacin): 15 milligrams (Note: A balanced B-complex is better than taking single B-vitamins)
>
> magnesium: 250–350 milligrams (this can be increased up to 3,000 milligrams with a nutritionist's recommendation)
>
> evening primrose oil: 1,000–1,500 milligrams GLA (best taken with zinc, omega-3 oils, vitamin C, B-complex)

vitamin C: 1–5 grams

zinc: 15 milligrams

B-complex (especially B_3 and B_6) in a balanced formula taken as directed
   on labels, with between 50–100 milligrams or more of each B vitamin
   (except B_{12}, which usually requires 300 micrograms a day)

Other Points

To improve cardiovascular stability and reduce background states of tension, begin a pattern of moderate exercise throughout the month.

Find creative ways that fit your budget and your time to reduce stress; avoid glare outdoors, get ample sleep, and take herbs to normalize the sex hormone cycle.

Biofeedback has been shown in many instances to improve a woman's own control over both vascular spasm and pain.

A significant minority of people with migraine are helped by applying moist heat to the head (even a hot shower), though this does not fit the logic of those whose pain results from over-dilated blood vessels.

Natural therapists can help address any food allergy or sensitivity, any deficiency of the enzyme MAO (monoamine oxidase), and platelet abnormalities.

Osteopathic or chiropractic alignment of cervical vertebrae and of the temperomandibular joint may help reduce tension in the head. Acupuncture and TENS (transcutaneous electrical stimulation) have also been helpful for some women, by changing the underlying imbalances or changing pain response.

PART THREE

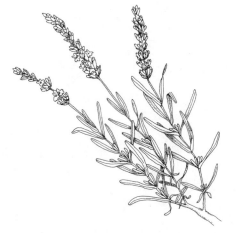

Abnormal Cell Growth

9

Fibroids

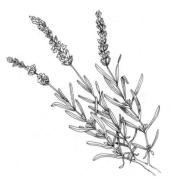

Definition

Fibroids are smooth-muscle tumors, called *leiomyomas* (*leio* = "smooth;" *my* = "muscle;" *oma* = "growth"). These benign growths of the uterine wall are stimulated by estrogen, growth hormone, blood sugar, and other cofactors. Fibroids are the most common benign tumors in western women today; one out of five women over age thirty-five has this condition, but many do not know it because most fibroids cause few symptoms.

The fibroid growths have the consistency of semi-solid protein—something like a hard-boiled egg. More muscular than "fibrous," fibroids are often felt upon routine gynecological examination. They range from the size of a pinhead to that of a football or a nine-month fetus.

Fibroids can be small or large, single or in clusters. Their rate of growth is usually slow, but these benign thickenings can grow quickly under stress. Sudden increases in estrogen levels also stimulate the growth of fibroids.

Symptoms and Signs

Fibroids can be quite large without causing any symptoms. Yet they can be quite small and still cause severe pelvic pain, heavy bleeding at menstruation, anemia, constipation, hemorrhoids, bladder problems (due to blockage and increased infections), or increased vulnerability to other diseases.

The most common symptom of any of these fibroid types is heavy periods, especially with the submucous (inside) and interstitial (middle layer) uterine locations. This is particularly true of women in later life, since most fibroids are slow-growing.

Another common symptom of large fibroids is a problem with bladder function: frequent urination or chronic bladder infections. The congestion in the pelvis may lead to more painful menstrual cramps and congestive dysmenorrhea, constipation, and varicose veins.

The uterus is a simple muscle that signals its discomfort with muscular contractions, causing one of the types of pain associated with fibroids. Painless fibroids may be found on routine examination, or after a number of heavy periods have led women to seek a diagnosis.

The symptom of heavy bleeding occurs partly because the fibroid makes the uterine lining thicken, creating more lining to slough off with each menstrual cycle.

A submucous fibroid (inside the uterine lining) may grow enough to poke down into the neck of the cervical opening from the womb to the vagina. Sometimes this is painful because it has a rich blood and nerve supply. The pain is often felt as central around the belly button, and may feel sharp, like muscle spasms or colic. These respond well to muscle-relaxing herbs, while a balanced formula over time gets to the cause.

The red or inflamed type of fibroid is of more immediate concern. It lets a woman know this with drill-like intensity. Herbal remedies recommended in this book are not narcotic or strong enough to completely suppress pain, so if they help, you'll be fine. If pain continues or gets worse, get a diagnosis and good care.

Fibroids can also cause some spotting between periods. This symptom requires a diagnosis before any reasonable treatment options can be decided upon. It may be nothing more than a symptom of tissue and hormonal imbalance; it may be something more.

Cause

Fibroids are common among western women between puberty and menopause. Near menopause, fibroids usually stop growing and even shrink, thanks to the natural drop in estrogen levels. If the fibroids are not too large or debilitating, it is usually safe to leave them in and let nature take its course. However, at any age herbs can help shrink fibroids.

Fibroids tend to occur more frequently in women without children. Heredity plays a role, as does nutrition. African-American women have a higher incidence of fibroids—three times as frequent as Caucasian, Latina, or Asian women.

Though there are many cofactors, the trigger for fibroids is hormonal. The smooth muscle of the womb is sensitive to hormones. It thickens under the influence of estrogen and human growth hormone. Progesterone has a stabilizing effect on the uterine lining. This sensitivity to hormones also depends on the health of the cells forming the womb.

This hormonal trigger to the growth of fibroids does not always explain the underlying cause of hormonal imbalance. Approaches based on hormones alone do not succeed as well as treatments that are suited to each woman's total health picture.

Conventional Medical Care

If you have a fibroid and surgery has been recommended, I encourage you to get second and third opinions, especially if you don't want a hysterectomy. Until recently, the medical establishment has resisted pressure from forward-thinking doctors to perform less drastic fibroid surgery. *Myomectomy* is the term for removing the fibroid without removing the whole uterus. This method is gaining acceptance as the more humane and medically appropriate treatment when surgery is unavoidable, especially for younger women who still want to have children.

Generally, surgery for fibroids is unnecessary during pregnancy. However, larger fibroids may interfere with pregnancy by signaling the body to spontaneously abort a fetus it cannot serve well enough with blood, oxygen, and nutrients.

Before any surgical intervention, herbs may assist the primary goal of removing a woman from immediate danger. Given adequate time, herbs may resolve the underlying imbalance and restore health. If surgery is required, herbal self-care will support health as a kind of "damage limitation" to offset trauma.

Hysterectomies have been the common conventional treatment for fibroids, but the current view is that surgery should not be performed unless fibroids are resistant to gentler treatment, or unless they are severe enough to threaten life. A more conservative approach than hysterectomy is to rule out malignant degeneration or threat to life, then make lifestyle changes designed to reduce fibroid size.

Herbal Treatment

If a woman chooses herbal therapy for fibroids, astringent, hormone-normalizing herbs can limit damage by shrinking overgrowth, lessening estrogen and other stimuli, assisting in bladder, bowel, and circulatory functions, and reducing heavy blood loss. This consistent therapy based on the woman, not the fibroid alone, allows one to reduce or clear fibroids over time.

If surgery is chosen, preventing regrowth with natural methods can improve a woman's quality of life.

There are seven herbal actions indicated for fibroids, and many possible herbal combinations. Each herb described here covers more than one of these actions, and their combination creates a synergistic effect.

Herbs that balance hormones, such as *Vitex agnus-castus* (chasteberry seed), promote healthy levels of progesterone; this and *Caulophyllum thalictroides* (blue cohosh root) appear to assist the body in reducing excess estrogen. Additional support from *Caulophyllum* includes its property of astringing uterine tissue, especially growths or wounds. *Anemone* (pasque flower herb) is also an astringent tonic; it modifies *Caulophyllum*'s stimulation of pelvic circulation.

Along with the aforementioned herbs, gentle pain-relieving herbs that have an affinity for women's reproductive pain are given, such as *Anemone pulsatilla* (pasque flower herb) and *Leonurus cardiaca* (motherwort herb).

Blood-sugar balancing herbs include bitters, such as *Verbena officinalis* (vervain herb), or endocrine remedies, such as *Oplopanax horridum* (devil's club root) and *Pfaffia paniculata* (suma).

Fresh extract of *Capsella bursa-pastoris* (shepherd's purse herb) is a circulatory stimulant that is also a uterine astringent. Antispasmodic *Viburnum prunifolium* (black haw bark) lessens cramping.

The treatment for fibroids has a lot in common with the herbal approach for congestive dysmenorrhea. Fibroids and painful periods often coexist, and it may sometimes be difficult to say which preceded the other.

Herbal Formula

Cimicifuga racemosa (black cohosh root)	2 ounces
Caulophyllum thalictroides (blue cohosh)	2 ounces
Vitex agnus-castus (chasteberry seed)	4 ounces
Viburnum prunifolium (black haw bark)	2 ounces
Verbena officinalis (vervain herb)	1 ounce
Leonurus cardiaca (motherwort herb)	2 ounces
Capsella bursa-pastoris (shepherd's purse herb)	3 ounces

This works well as a combined tincture of alcohol-based or glycerin extracts. If fresh shepherd's purse tincture is not readily available (see "Resources"), it may be replaced in this formula by an equal amount of *Vinca major* or *Vinca minor* (periwinkle herb).

You may take fresh shepherd's purse extract on its own as needed to control excess bleeding. You can then make tea or capsules of the other herbs to be taken throughout the month. Shepherd's purse does not work well as a dried herb in tea.

Even without shepherd's purse, this formula does not taste good as a tea. It is bitter, but if you need it your taste buds will get used to it.

Tea may be made more tasty with the addition of:

Rubus idaeus (raspberry leaf)	5 ounces
Melissa officinalis (lemon balm leaf)	5 ounces

The preparation is standard; the dose for the tea is 4 cups a day (16 fluid ounces), hot or cold. Continue for at least three months or three complete menstrual cycles. Best results are obtained by taking the herbs for six months to a year, since the slow-growing fibroids usually reflect a more long-standing imbalance than actual symptoms show.

Though a general maxim in natural therapy is to take herbs consistently at least one month for every year that a condition has been present, in the case of fibroids treatment may run longer. Though herbs may quickly relieve symptoms, it takes time for the body to change its response to stress.

If you become bored with taking the same tea or tincture every day for six to twelve months, you may replace raspberry leaf and peppermint with fennel seeds, star anise, or hibiscus flowers to taste. Try tincture diluted in black cherry juice instead of water. Or try disguising tincture in a tea made with licorice root and orange peel.

If severe pain is a significant problem, it must be diagnosed and the cause addressed. Meanwhile, for a stronger muscle relaxing and analgesic formula add to the above Herbal Formula:

Viburnum opulus (cramp bark)	2 ounces
Passiflora incarnata (passionflower herb)	2 ounces

One of the best herbs for fibroids and other reproductive imbalance, *Chamaelirium luteum* (false unicorn root), has been endangered until recently. Other tonic herbs for the uterus include the endangered *Hydrastis canadensis* (goldenseal root) and *Trillium spp.* (Bethroot). Buy these at an herb shop only if their supply is organically grown rather than collected in the wild.

Nutrition

Choose whole foods, with generous amounts of raw fruits, grains and vegetables. Avoid excess caffeine and sugar intake. Caffeine is linked to a rise in estrogen levels and nervous irritability; reducing it even a little will improve your overall health if you wish to clear fibroids naturally. Eat complex carbohydrates, balanced with dark green vegetables and lean protein.

Especially good vegetables to choose from three times a week are liver-friendly foods: carrots, beets, greens, parsley, watercress, sprouts, spinach, celery, dandelion and collard greens, kale, sea vegetables (seaweed), plus one clove of garlic daily. Cooked vegetables in soup are recommended two nights a week during cold weather; lighter broths or raw salads with sprouts during warm weather are recommended three times a week or more as desired.

When the symptom of fatigue from fibroids gains on you, you can get extra energy by nibbling on five to ten organic pecans or almonds a day or a teaspoon of local bee pollen.

If fibroids cause heavy bleeding and anemia, eat twenty raisins a day or 1 tablespoon of blackstrap molasses and read Chapter 7: Anemia.

Drink at least eight glasses of water a day.

Other Points

Exercise moderately to increase pelvic circulation, but don't overdo it.

Castor oil packs are a standard natural treatment for reducing fibroids. They are described under Preparations (Chapter 2) in the section on Oils.

Fibroids cause fatigue. Natural remedies assist the body to clear the cause, but it is important to allow time for recuperation during this self-cleansing process. Rest a lot. Instead of fighting the fatigue take naps and your energy will return sooner.

10

Ovarian Cysts

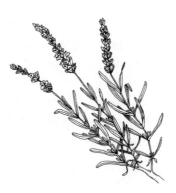

Definition

Ovarian cysts are usually benign, and they respond well to alternative treatment. (A cyst is a closed sac usually filled with fluid or semisolid material.) As many as ninety-five percent of all ovarian cysts are not serious. They can occur at any time between puberty and menopause, including during pregnancy. Common follicular cysts often go away without any treatment in two or three months.

Ovarian cysts are commonly either follicular cysts or lutein cysts. Lutein cysts develop either from granulosa or theca cells of the corpus luteum. Polycystic ovarian disease (PCOD) occurs when several cysts develop simultaneously.

With the follicular type of ovarian cyst, the follicle may grow too big under the influence of estrogen, adrenaline, and other hormones.

Symptoms and Signs

Common symptoms of large ovarian cysts include mild pelvic discomfort or pain, low back ache, pain with sexual intercourse, or irregular bleeding. These also occur when there are several small cysts. When there are follicular cysts on one ovary, a follicle may not get big enough to be painful every month. Symptoms can be sporadic, with some cycles relatively pain-free.

Ovarian cysts may be on one or both ovaries, resulting either in painful ovulation every month, or pain on different sides in different months. Other symptoms include late periods, irregular cycles, or heavy bleeding.

Because a large cyst can rupture, causing dangerous internal bleeding, severe or chronic pain must be diagnosed before beginning natural treatment. Warning signs include a suddenly painful or bloated belly, fever, or rigid abdominal muscles with pain. The good news is that once a cyst ruptures, it usually does not grow back.

Polycystic ovarian disease is part of a larger endocrine imbalance, usually causing anovulatory (heavy) periods without ovulation, weight gain, and facial hair growth.

As long as ovarian cysts come and go, they are changing, so it is possible for the self-healing impulse of the body to change ovaries back to a healthy function and size. If symptoms disappear when a woman is on the contraceptive pill, it is worth trying natural herbal hormone balancers, which may clear up the imbalance without the side effects caused by this form of birth control.

Cause

The two weeks leading up to ovulation are the *follicular* phase of the menstrual cycle. If the follicular phase is long, estrogen builds up and sometimes causes the developing follicle to get very large. If a woman's body doesn't reabsorb this with normal immune and reproductive function, this large follicle may fill with fluid and persist as a follicular cyst. Normally the follicle shrinks during the luteal phase (second half) of the menstrual cycle. A swollen ovarian follicle may hurt, and may be felt on examination. Some women can feel the follicular cysts burst, sometimes painfully, upon release of the egg. The follicle may get as large as two inches in diameter when its capsule bursts, but it might feel much larger. When in doubt, get a diagnosis from a qualified practitioner. An enlarged ovary is usually felt during an exam, but a small ovarian cyst may cause no symptoms. Since it is easiest to feel a cyst before ovulation, plan appointments then or when in pain to gain the most information.

If follicular cysts continue into menopause, they will be stimulated by the normal surge of follicle-stimulating hormone (FSH) and luteinizing hormone (LH) that occurs at that time. Follicular cysts then secrete an excess of estrogen. The conservative approach is to wait a few months and see if the body handles this on its own. Alternatively, an herbal approach combines hepatics, alteratives, hormonal normalizers, and nervines (see Herbal Formula III: Perimenopause, in the "Herbal Treatment" section of this chapter).

Conventional Medical Care

Usually there is no treatment recommended since follicular cysts tend to go away on their own in a couple of months. Otherwise, if pain interferes with a woman's quality of life, progesterone or other hormone therapy is used to reestablish the hormonal cycle of ovulation. Birth control pills may help shrink ovarian cysts.

During pregnancy, the treatment for granulosa-lutein cysts is to reduce symptoms with mild anti-inflammatories or analgesics since these usually disappear by the end of pregnancy. They rarely require surgery. If they are caused by a growth that produces hormones, removal of the growth is normal.

Treatment of PCOD is varied; it depends on the underlying cause of the continuing overgrowth of cysts on the ovary. Sometimes cysts that do not go away on their own in one or two cycles are removed and studied to help with diagnosis. Sometimes the approach is to induce ovulation with synthetic progesterone or other drugs, or to surgically remove part of the over-functioning but inefficient ovary, along with treating the endocrine disorder contributing to PCOD.

Herbal Treatment

Herbs, especially in combination with supportive nutrition and perhaps some form of counseling, are safe and effective for women who have this painful but common condition. Herbal care can help a woman move through this time more easily, and often more quickly. For cysts that do not resolve easily, herbs still have a tremendous role to play in restoring ovarian harmony.

Once it has been determined that the cyst is benign, the objective of holistic treatment is to restore function via hormonal balance and tissue health. This is done by reducing excess estrogen in the follicular phase, while balancing excess progesterone from the corpus luteum during the second half of the cycle. No research has been done to show that herbs work the way they are described here, but results in women clients lead herbalists to hypothesize that the herbs have hormone-balancing effects along with their known tissue-toning properties related to self-repair.

Traditionally, herbalists choose astringent anti-inflammatories to decrease the size of cysts and the enlarged and inflamed ovary. Antispasmodics are used to decrease tenderness. The use of herbs to support the next natural ovulation may work through roundabout mechanisms to establish endocrine self-regulation, rather than by stimulating the ovarian clock to ovulate on cue. Though the herb *Vitex* (chasteberry) is said to strengthen the corpus luteum by stimulating LH from the pituitary, some herbalists have paradoxically found these medicinal herb seeds helpful in clearing PCOD in combination with other herbs. This makes it difficult to assess whether the *Vitex* is overridden by other herbs in a formula, or if it has a balancing effect rather than an automatically stimulating effect through the pituitary on ovarian function. PCOD is associated with high LH and low FSH.

Herbal Formula I: Bleeding Through Ovulation

Caulophyllum thalictroides (blue cohosh root)	3 ounces
Cimicifuga racemosa (black cohosh root)	3 ounces
Achillea millefolium (yarrow flower)	1 ounce
Dioscorea villosa (wild yam root)	2 ounces
Viburnum prunifolium (black haw bark)	2 ounces
Carduus or *Silybum marianum* (milk thistle seed)	3 ounces

Tea, capsules, or tincture—all are fine with this formula. For tea, use 1½ ounces of herb mixture in 3 to 4 cups of water; for flavor, add herbs such as cinnamon or hibiscus to taste. Strain tea; drink 3 cups a day, hot or cold.

If you are combining tinctures or extracts, take 1 teaspoon of the mixture in water three times a day.

For capsules, grind the herbs separately and mix well; fill #00 capsules and take two capsules with a glass of water three times a day with meals. If more information is needed, see Chapter 2: Herbal Preparation.

Take consistently during the first two weeks of each cycle for at least three periods or three months. Six to nine months on the herbal formulas is preferable.

If irregular and long cycles accompany cysts, add 2 ounces of *Angelica sinensis* (dong quai).

Herbal Formula II: Ovulation to Bleeding

Vitex agnus-castus (chasteberry seed)	3 ounces
Cimicifuga racemosa (black cohosh root)	3 ounces
Taraxacum officinalis (dandelion root and leaf, equal parts)	2 ounces
Dioscorea villosa (wild yam root)	2 ounces
Viburnum prunifolium (black haw bark)	2 ounces

Prepare and take as described for the Bleeding-Through-Ovulation formula.

Ovarian cysts at menopause may result in higher estrogen levels, but even though *Cimicifuga* (black cohosh root) is considered to promote estrogen it also seems to reduce LH levels. It is also specific for reducing hot flashes and irritability. This means that it often benefits the woman with cysts during or near menopause. Because perimenopausal cycles are more irregular or even absent, one formula only is taken through the month:

Herbal Formula III: Perimenopause

Berberis aquifolium (Oregon grape root)	1 ounce
Smilax ornata (sarsaparilla root)	2 ounces

| *Cimicifuga racemosa* (black cohosh root) | 2 ounces |
| *Scutellaria lateriflora* (skullcap herb) | 3 ounces |

Prepare and take as described for the Bleeding-Through-Ovulation formula.

Nutrition

Avoid alcohol, red meat, carbonated beverages, caffeine, and processed or refined foods. Increase your intake of raw fruits and vegetables, limit excess carbohydrates, and have only one to two servings of complex carbohydrate daily (not too much whole wheat bread, pasta, or brown rice). Simple measures truly show best effects. Natural treatments for cysts work better when women are enjoying some high-quality protein (vegetable or animal: lean fish, beans, and grains) in a whole-food context.

Other Points

The relationship between mind, body, and emotion has been found to be important to immune function and overall health. Some women report that, with a qualified therapist whom they trust, counseling, hypnotherapy, and positive imagery have been effective. While it is becoming more common to speak of these relationships in the mainstream Western culture, many women still "skip" this part of self-healing. Being too busy for such "extra" work on one's health may be part of our dis-ease. Studies on visualization, relaxation, and clearing old emotional traumas consistently demonstrate that these nonphysical healing methods always have value. The key is to follow through on one's inner promptings to engage in the type of "inner work" that makes sense to each woman.

11

Cervical Dysplasia
INFLAMMATION, EROSION, AND EVERSION

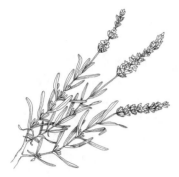

Definition

Dysplasia means dysfunctional, or abnormal, cell growth. Having abnormal cells on the cervix is not the same as having cancer. A lot of panic accompanies common misunderstandings about this part of a woman's body and the medicalization of women's bodies.

The surface of the cervix is covered with a type of cell called *epithelial* cells. Like the cells lining the inside of the mouth, these cells are accustomed to some friction and being worn down, sloughed off, and replaced frequently.

Inflammation of the cervix is called *cervicitis*. Chronic (long-lasting) forms of cervicitis are associated with *eversion* (when the cells on the cervix seem to turn inside out) or with ulcerative lesions from Herpes Simplex Virus II. Chronic cervicitis is usually inadequately treated acute cervicitis that recurs.

Though it is inexact to interchange the terms "dysplasia" (abnormal cell growth) and "cervicitis" (inflamed cervix), these are often lumped together with other nonmalignant cell changes on the surface of the cervix. *Hyperplasia* simply means that the cells are growing a little too fast and too thick, as if they are responding to repeated irritation. This is the way the cervix cushions itself against excessive impact, chemical or physical. *Neoplasia* simply means new cell growth and does not in itself indicate cancerous growth.

Symptoms and Signs

Cervicitis creates a clear, persistent discharge from the vagina, especially in chronic cases. "Persistent" means that the discharge doesn't clear up soon or comes back more than once; this requires a checkup. In acute cervicitis, discharge may be foul-smelling, greenish, or blood-stained, any of which must be cultured to determine the cause. This discharge may create itching or burning anywhere from the cervix to the outer vulva. On examination, the cervix appears swollen and red (see Chapter 18: Vaginitis for information relating to reproductive infections).

The surface of the cervix that faces downward into the vagina is normally covered with epithelial cells shaped like flat tiles stacked in a few layers. Under these layers are "vascular beds" of many tiny blood vessels, supplying the area with blood and nutrients. But with chronic infection or any ongoing inflammation, these tile-shaped surface cells become swollen and easily irritated. Their fragility may cause sexual intercourse to be painful, and there may be spotty bleeding after sex.

The epithelial cells that line the os are shaped like tall columns standing side by side. Chronic inflammation of these cells causes eversion—a condition in which the cells start to turn outward onto the downward-facing surface of the cervix. These tall, thin cells are not designed to handle friction or impact, so when they are irritated by sexual intercourse, chemicals in tampons, or other trauma, the surface gets inflamed and painful. This leads to more spotting, likelihood of secondary infection, scarring, and rapid regrowth of new cells.

New cells born into this stressed tissue are not always healthy. Often nutritional and hormonal states are out of balance at the same time. If there has been antibiotic treatment there may be immune-system breakdown. Stress has a variety of effects that slow self-repair. The fragile surface is vulnerable to *erosion*, in which the cell gets damaged because it is positioned in the wrong place.

All unexplained bleeding must be traced to its cause rather than generally attributed to "stress." Once the cause is known, natural treatments may end a vicious cycle of stress, tissue breakdown, and abnormal cell development.

Cause

During periods of high stress or illness, increased cellular activity shows up as a rapid turnover of cells. Of all the many dividing cells, some can divide with little mistakes in their lineup of proteins, possibly leading to abnormal cells. Our immune system is designed to recognize, destroy, and mop up "wrong" cells, given a fighting chance. Also, this means that improving our response to stress can impact our cervical cells and the way they divide.

Cervical diseases reflect poor diet, other kinds of disease, hormonal imbalance, stress, and, yes, sometimes cancer.

A common condition strongly associated with dysplasia and cervical cancer is infection with Human Papilloma Virus (HPV, responsible for genital warts). But having this sexually transmitted disease is not a certain route to cancer, as many women fear. The birth control pill is also linked to cervical cancer, as are smoking and folic acid deficiency.

Sudden (or "acute") cervicitis is often due to such infections as the common *Neisseria* (gonorrhea).

Cervicitis is just one kind of pelvic inflammatory disease (PID) in which any part of the female reproductive tract can be inflamed (causes range from gonorrhea to IUDs). Untreated, PID can lead to infertility and abnormal vaginal bleeding. It can endanger pregnancies, increase vulnerability to other infective organisms, or cause degeneration of tissues.

Risk factors for cervical erosion or abnormal cell growth include:

- sexual activity at an early age
- multiple sex partners
- STDs (sexually transmitted diseases: HPV, herpes, chlamydia, etc.)
- PID and other infections
- D&Cs
- multiple therapeutic abortions
- IUDs (intrauterine devices for contraception)
- hormonal imbalance
- DES (diethylstilbestrol) use, especially if by a woman's mother
- oral contraceptives
- synthetic hormones such as xenoestrogens (foreign or "strange" estrogens) in the environment
- carcinogens including dioxin
- smoking and secondhand smoke
- high-risk jobs, including sex work
- cervical cancer or partners with penile or cervical cancer
- vitamin deficiencies (B_{12}, C, folic acid)
- stress

Conventional Medical Care

Conventional medical treatments for dysplasia aggressively hunt out and burn off (cauterization) or freeze the affected cervix (cryosurgery), often without addressing the cause of abnormal cell development. Conventional treatment may even aggravate or complicate the underlying cause of abnormal cell growth.

Cervical dysplasia has become a scary condition because the Western medical view is that it requires constant scrutiny or it will become cancer. In defense of allopaths, once a practitioner has seen what can go wrong, it is only human to see that worrisome situation everywhere until proven otherwise. But this is not always good medicine.

The medical view of a woman's body isn't too helpful, either; it is seen as inconsequential to burn and scar the narrow portal between the "entry halls" of the vagina and a woman's uterus—the inner sanctum of life. Women are more than a walking cancer risk. It is insane to remove tissue that is doing its job by sending distress signals to a woman to make her pay attention to her total health.

Occasionally, surgery can be life-saving; let it be done with genuine need only. But even when surgery is called for, if the underlying causes are not addressed, abnormal cells may simply grow again anyway.

Pap Testing

An understanding of Pap smears is useful for every woman, and can be especially helpful when using herbs to treat cervical changes. The test, developed by Dr. George Papinocolaou, identifies cell changes that are related to infection or estrogen levels, and detects a high percentage of cancers. The test involves looking at endocervical cells that are a part of the cervix lining and the superficial (visible) cells of the cervix, which are scraped off (it's not painful) and analyzed. Samples from the vaginal walls may also be taken. It is for screening purposes and does not diagnose a condition.

Frequent Pap testing "just to be sure" is of debatable value. There are those who believe that we find what we are looking for, so only have Pap tests redone after major health changes or with routine health screening as needed.

The interpretation of the Pap smear is based on the changes seen in the cells. False results are a problem if women douche or use vaginal treatments within twenty-four hours of the test.

Class I, a "normal" smear, shows mature epithelial cells. Class II, "mild dysplasia," is indicated by a mixture of mature and immature cells. The higher the percentage of immature cells, the more fragile the surface of the cervix. Even normal impact may cause these fragile cells to break, leading to bleeding, pain, or infection.

Class III, Pap result—"moderate"—is more open to interpretation. In this case, the lower third of the epithelium is abnormal; this condition is still categorized as self-limiting, meaning that it usually goes back to normal.

Whether women choose to treat this symptom naturally or not, ignoring moderate dysplasia is not recommended by health care providers of any belief system. Depending on how the cells respond to the chosen method of care, the dysplasia may progress to "severe," in which two-thirds or more of the epithelial cells show abnormal overgrowth.

Class IV, the next stage—"carcinoma in situ"—sounds terrifying, but it means that pre-invasive patches of abnormal cells are in place. They may become carcinomas, and they have not spread. This stage is also called "CIN," which stands for "cervical intraepithelial neoplasia." The scrapings of the cervix show that a full thickness of the epithelial cell layer contains abnormal cells. They can be removed or changed allopathically, or with effort over time using remedies that affect the cervix from the inside as well as the outside of the body.

CIN is not as much a cancerous condition as it is a late-stage warning bell to change a precancerous condition into wholeness. When pre-invasive cancer is caught early and treated thoroughly, it can be cleared in seventy-five to ninety percent of women. Women may prefer to wait and monitor their return to wholeness over two to six months instead of reacting with fear. When invasive cancer is ruled out, the conventional treatment is cryotherapy (freezing off the abnormal cervical cells) or conization (obliterating the cells by grinding away the surface of the cervix). If these methods work, natural therapies have a chance to help, as there is time while monitoring continues.

"Invasive carcinoma" means that abnormal cells can be seen extending deeper into the basement membrane below the surface cells (epithelium). From here, abnormal cells have the opportunity to spread to other places in the pelvis or, through the lymphatic circulation, to anywhere in the body. But it usually stays local for a considerable length of time—long enough for conventional or natural treatments to have a chance at restoring tissue integrity. This is usually *squamous cell carcinoma*; occasionally invasive cancer is *adenocarcinoma*. When squamous cell carcinoma is responsibly treated with natural treatments, the success rate is similar to that of methods such as radiation plus surgery, or for surgical removal of just the cancer and affected lymph nodes. Surgery is no guarantee of avoiding malignancy, though some women are pressured by their physicians to go this route.

A final note about using the Pap smear to monitor a condition: The standard recommendation is to scrape the cervix or even cut out a little wedge for diagnosis (colposcopy), temporarily leaving a red, inflamed cervix. It may require up to three months of rest, nutrition, and general wellness for a woman's body to replace damaged tissue with a layer of mature, normal cells. But fear of cancer and its spread through the lymph nodes requires that practitioners retest patients every month or six weeks. This seems like a good way to keep finding abnormally inflamed cells. Because cervical cancer is one of the most common gynecological cancers in North America, monitoring is wise, but improving all known areas to avoid unnecessary risk is the most reliable route to whole health.

Herbal Treatment

Abnormal cell growth on the cervix does not always require the heavy-handed tools of allopathy. In herbal medicine, impaired cellular function is seen as caused by an unhealthy internal environment. With depressed immunity, the usual means of curtailing or eliminating abnormal cells is weakened. To correct this, herbs are given to cleanse, strengthen, and support the liver, immune system, lymphatic circulation, and nervous and reproductive systems. General circulation, kidney, and lung function may enter the treatment picture with women whose health history indicates a need for this.

The natural approach is to apply herbs to an inflamed, infected, or eroded surface of the cervix. This may be all that is needed for the self-healing, self-organizing principle to return cervical cells to homeostasis—a dynamic balance of health. Such herbal applications may be also combined with internal treatment, as described in this section.

The os will rearrange its "tiles and columns" to their own appropriate locations whenever possible. Herbs do not cause this healing; they help the body's self-healing principles of cell repair. In addition, high quality nutrition over several weeks or months provides other ingredients for self-healing.

Herbalists first rule out pathology, usually by working with licensed practitioners, before treating the less deadly and far more common disturbances of natural function. Rebalancing function is what herbs do best, whether reducing heavy menstrual flow, disinfecting reddened tissues, or stimulating natural immune-system defenses against chronic subclinical infection. In the case of cervical cell changes, all these functions are improved by a regular ticking of the ovarian clock, so hormonal normalizing herbs add to the good "tone" of the cells forming the cervix.

The objective of holistic treatment is to normalize mucous membranes of the vaginal and cervical tissues, balance hormones, and restore cellular integrity to new epithelium. A combination of herbal infusions used as douches will relieve symptoms of inflammation or bleeding. Once causes have been identified, internal (oral) herbal alteratives and hormonal and reproductive-tissue tonics are used.

The most important herbal actions for a woman with cervical dysplasia are astringents with an affinity for the reproductive tissues, such as *Vinca spp.* (periwinkle leaf) and *Alchemilla vulgaris* (lady's mantle herb), and antimicrobial vulneraries, such as *Calendula* (calendula flowers) or *Hydrastis canadensis* (goldenseal root).

Though the plant is overharvested, endangered, and generally overused by the natural healing community, my favorite herb for use in dysplasia is still *Hydrastis canadensis* (goldenseal). There are times like this when no other treatment does so much, and very small amounts of the root powder in tea or tincture can be effective. Applied locally (to heal the cervix) and taken orally, goldenseal is an astringent that disinfects and tones the mucous membranes (vaginal, cervical, uterine, and other). Furthermore, goldenseal taken orally is a potent bitter tonic for liver function that helps hormone balance, immune-system function, and the central digestive tract. These benefits extend to the blood, lungs, and skin. For these reasons, though goldenseal can sometimes be replaced with *Anemopsis californica* (yerba mansa root) or *Berberis aquifolium* (Oregon grape root), it is included in the formula for cervical dysplasia.

Hormonal tonic herbs that contain phytoestrogens (plant hormones) are not necessarily contraindicated when estrogen-dependent growth presents a health risk. There is debate and contradictory experimental evidence about this. Naturally occurring plant hormones called phytosterols appear to interact with steroidal receptors to improve negative feedback loops and the body's own control over levels of hormones. Herbs do not have the same effect on our tissues as the estrogen that is given as a prescription drug, the birth control pill, or hormone replacement therapy. Two popular hormone balancing herbs with phytoestrogenic activity are *Angelica sinensis* (dong quai root) and *Glycyrrhiza glabra* (licorice root).

A holistic approach takes time to explain, since we give herbs to each woman; we can't give herbs to the cervix. The following herbs, and the later suggestions for nutrition, however, are a great starting point.

Herbal Formula I

Hydrastis canadensis (goldenseal root)	1 ounce
Smilax ornata (sarsaparilla root)	2 ounces
Thuja occidentalis (cedar or thuja leaf)	1 ounce
Calendula officinalis (calendula flower)	3 ounces
Caulophyllum thalictroides (blue cohosh)	2 ounces
Verbena officinalis (vervain herb)	1 ounce

Due to the number of herbs and their flavor, this is best taken as a combination of tinctures or extracts (alcohol or alcohol-free). Depending on availability, *Thuja* may be replaced by *Smilax* (sarsaparilla root) or *Echinacea spp.* (root, seed).

Combine tinctures in the proportions given (or, to make a compound tincture, see Chapter 2: Herbal Preparation). The dose is one teaspoon in water or herb tea, three times a day, for a minimum of two months; four months is better, even when symptoms may be absent.

Alternatively, you may take the ground herbs in two #00 capsules with a large glass of water, diluted juice, or herb tea, three times a day.

Eating a little something with capsules or the strong-tasting tincture allows stomach enzymes to digest the herbs well. This may help if your stomach is sensitive, but taking this formula with food is not usually necessary.

Since cervical dysplasia may both cause and be caused by emotional stress, if chronic or severe stress is a concern, add 1 ounce each of *Scutellaria* (skullcap herb) and *Pfaffia paniculata* (suma root).

If there has been liver disease from travel or exposure to harmful substances, add liver support and cleansing with 1 ounce of *Silybum* or *Carduus* (milk thistle seed) or *Taraxacum* (dandelion root).

If dysplasia is associated with an infection of the reproductive tract, especially if you are taking antibiotics, add acidophilus and live-culture yogurts to your diet. When the nasturtium *(Tropaeolum officinale)* is in season, eat 1/6 ounce of fresh leaves and the yellow-orange flowers tossed into a salad every few days, or as desired. Though it is hot to the taste, the peppery vegetable contains many nutrients for promoting circulation and healing. This beautiful herb grows easily from seed in a pot on a sunny counter or window box on the sill.

If you want alterative herbs that are considered anticancer (antineoplastic), add 2 ounces of *Viola odorata* (sweet violet) and/or *Trifolium pratense* (red clover), and 1 ounce of *Arctium lappa* (burdock root).

If dysplasia is associated with use of the birth control pill, consider alternative contraception and then add 2 ounces *Vitex agnus-castus* (chasteberry seed). If you continue to use the birth control pill, don't add *Vitex* but do add 2 ounces of *Hydrastis canadensis* (goldenseal) and 4 parts of *Althaea officinalis* (marshmallow).

External Herbal Therapies

With a little willingness, herbal preparations for vaginal use can be made at home. They are effective, but their preparation may seem time-consuming at first. They may also feel awkward to use at first.

Douches   Healthy vaginas do not require douching. Overuse of even natural douches can cause problems. However, when the cervix is inflamed or exhibiting stress at the cellular level, as in dysplasia, gentle medicinal herb douches are part of a total approach. Herbal douches used as recommended here do not strip away normal bacteria or secretions. They have a reputation for cleansing the tissue, reducing bleeding, and strengthening the cervix. These douches can be used twice weekly for up to three months.

A wheatgrass douche is my first choice. Use plain wheatgrass juice if it is available fresh; you can easily grow and juice it at home. Add 1 ounce of juice per 6 ounces of sterile water (boiled, filtered, or distilled). If wheatgrass isn't an option, try one or more of the following herbs.

Vaginal Herbal Formula I: External Use as Douche

Vinca major or minor (periwinkle leaf)	4 ounces
Hydrastis canadensis (goldenseal root)	1 ounce
Hydrocotyle asiatica (gotu kola herb)	1 ounce
Althaea officinalis (marshmallow root)	3 ounces

Grind the herbs in a blender or coffee grinder. Follow the preparation instructions for an infusion, but make it double strength by using only 4 ounces of water. Strain well and let it cool to a comfortable temperature.

Alternatively, use tinctures (in the same proportions, using teaspoonfuls instead of ounces of herb); mix the four tinctures with one cup of boiled (sterilized) water that has cooled to a comfortable temperature.

Introduce the herbal formula into the vagina using a douche bag; hold it inside for five minutes or more, with your feet elevated (sit on the toilet with your legs propped up on a footstool, or relax in a warm bath with your feet resting comfortably on the edge of the tub). After five minutes, let the herbal liquid run out of you. It is not necessary to follow the douche with plain water; the herbs have an anti-inflammatory and vulnerary effect. Repeat two to five times a week, depending on available time or the severity of the dysplasia. Continue for a minimum of four weeks for up to four months, with one or more checkups to monitor cervical changes.

The periwinkle in this formula is *Vinca major* or *Vinca minor*. These two interchangeable species are the common European and American garden vine with larger (*major*) or smaller (*minor*) blue flowers.

A more widely known periwinkle used in herbal medicine is neither closely related nor similar in properties: *Canthareus roseus*, or Madagascan periwinkle, contains alkaloids that are useful in the treatment of childhood leukemia. This herb was researched intensively by drug companies; it is also endangered now. Some bright lights went on in the FDA's collective mind when it tried to take the common Euro-American periwinkle off the market because it confused its properties with those of *Canthareus*, apparently believing that any herb with anticancer potential must be a dangerous plant. This led to public misinformation that is only slowly clearing up now. The common periwinkle is available; used as directed, it is a safe astringent tonic.

Sometimes dysplasia responds best to changing treatment, as if the cervix gets bored with just one formula over time. Vaginal Herbal Formula II, with the antiviral calendula and thuja oils, has a different action and can be substituted or used as an alternate every other week.

Vaginal Herbal Formula II: External Use as Douche

water (sterilized)	1 cup, warm but not hot
calendula oil	1 ounce
vitamin E oil	15 drops
thuja essential oil	15 drops
Optional:	
geranium essential oil	4–6 drops
blue chamomile essential oil	4–6 drops

Dilute the combined oils in one cup of warm water, and shake or whisk the oils and water well. Insert the liquid gently into vagina with a douche bag; hold in for five minutes with your feet elevated, if that's comfortable (see directions for Vaginal Herbal Formula I). Using optional oils makes this a deliciously aromatic douche with added anti-inflammatory action. Including the essential oils makes this a more expensive formula. Essential oils are available at retail stores or from suppliers listed in the Appendix.

One advantage to making this formula with essential oils is its aromatherapy value: The scent makes the act of taking your medicine an esthetic pleasure. Enjoying your nightly "medicine" is especially important when stress and body image have made a negative impact on a woman's health.

The atrociously named but successful Vaginal Depletion Pack is the most complicated recipe in this chapter. It was developed by the Eclectic Physicians, a large group of American doctors who used herbs during the nineteenth century, and whose practitioners still exist today. The primary application of this formula handed out at feminist self-help groups for the last several years is in treating cervical erosion and other conditions that cause abnormal Pap smears. It seems to work in part because the herbs act locally as antimicrobials. Little published research has been done to determine the actual mechanism of its efficacy. It is possible to prepare at home using this recipe, or it can be purchased from suppliers listed in the Appendix.

Vaginal Depletion Pack

MgSO$_4$ (anhydrous magnesium sulfate)	8 ounces
glycerin (same as vegetable glycerin, glycerol)	4–6 ounces
ti tree essential oil	¼ ounce
thuja essential oil	½ ounce
bitter orange essential oil	¼ ounce

goldenseal tincture	½ ounce
Vita Minerals 120 (iron sulfate solution)	1 ounce

1. Pour the $MgSO_4$ into a wide-mouthed 16-ounce glass container (with tight-fitting lid) until it is half full.
2. Add glycerin until soupy.

    Note: Mix vigorously after each of the following steps, or the solution won't be usable.

3. Add essential oils.
4. Add goldenseal tincture.
5. Add iron sulfate solution.

Stir occasionally over the next two to three hours, until the mixture has a thick, tar-like consistency, then store in a tightly sealed container in a cool place. Stir once every week if not used regularly. It keeps indefinitely with proper storage and occasional stirring.

Now fold a piece of cotton cloth, ½ by 2 by 3 inches long, lengthwise into a tube. Tie one end with a 4-inch cotton string or dental floss, leaving a long "tail." Put 1 tablespoon of the formula into the untied end of the cotton tube. Using a speculum (a plastic or metal instrument used to examine the cervix; available at women's health clinics, with use instructions), expose the cervix; open the speculum wide enough to insert the pack. Slide the pack, formula-end first, tightly up against the cervix (uterine forceps can be used to hold the pack in place as speculum is removed). Leave the string exposed for later removal of the herb pack. Leave the pack in for twenty-four hours, then remove it by pulling the string. Twenty-four hours after removal, use a mild apple cider vinegar douche (1 teaspoon of vinegar diluted in 8 ounces of water).

This pack may be used any time except during menstruation. The best time for application is right after menses or during ovulation.

Typically, women will notice an increase in drainage after use. If there is burning while the pack is inserted, remove it and douche with the mild vinegar solution right away. Within a few days of application, the cervix will have a red, eroded appearance where cells have sloughed off. This typically heals in seven to ten days. Results of a follow-up Pap smear should begin improving after four to six applications; more advanced dysplasia may take longer.

During external (vaginal) treatment, Pap smears should be repeated no more than once a month, allowing at least ten days after each application to ensure adequate healing time for reliable tests. Otherwise the raw, red surface of new cells may be interpreted as a worsening, instead of an improving, cervical tissue sample. Most often "inconclusive" results lead to more testing and plenty of nail-biting.

The external (vaginal) approach is aided by nutritional changes, internal herbal therapy, patience, and a great deal of self-love.

Nutrition

Avoid excess alcohol, caffeine, high-fat or fried foods, hot spices, pungent foods such as pickles and preserved meats, acrid foods, red meat, heavy or hard-to-digest food, preservatives, sugars, flavorings or chemicals, and overeating in general.

Add cleansing raw foods, vegetable juices, non-mucus-producing foods (fresh fruits, vegetables, brown rice), and high-quality bioavailable protein (lean fish, beans, and grains) in small amounts. Avoid dairy, oats, bread, and sugar.

Supplements

I recommend the following quantities daily:

folic acid: 5 milligrams twice a day for three months

vitamin C: 3,000 milligrams or more, with bioflavonoids

vitamin A: 60,000 IU daily for two months, then 25,000 IU

selenium: 200 milligrams

germanium: 60 milligrams GE

antioxidants: vitamins A, C, and E (internally and externally)

Germanium is a wound-healing nutrient that is also considered antineoplastic. It is found in high concentrations in garlic and suma root.

Other Points

Meditation, imagery, relaxation, counseling techniques, and lifestyle changes can all help to reduce stress. Women with a diagnosis of severe cervical cell changes have been known to meditate for twenty minutes a day for eight weeks, without changing their diet or lifestyle or taking herbs, then get a retest that shows a cervix on the mend.

This is not to deny the importance of identifying true indications of precancer. Holistic care includes eating wisely and taking herbs when there is time for a change, but it also means seeing a conventional gynecologist when there is no time for a remedy such as meditation or herbal treatment.

Look again at the list of risk factors in the "Cause" section of this chapter. What does it tell us? Not that sex is bad. Sex is sacred—a metaphor of greater unity in life and conscious surrender to love. But when we treat our sexuality or our life in a profane way, the result is disease.

The cure for dysplasia and cervical cancer is not more Pap tests for earlier detection. Digging out cancerous cells without changing their reasons for mutation is not the cure either. Following removal of cancerous cells, responsible treatment with appropriate medicine may include herbs or conventional drugs. But integrated medicine always includes bringing one's beliefs about sexuality and self into harmony with one's physical expression in the world.

Give it time. Keep monitoring progress, but expect to see healing.

12

Endometriosis

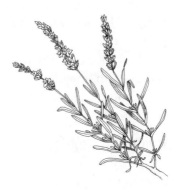

Definition

The lining of the uterus is made up of a cell layer called the *endometrium* (*endo*, "inside"; *metrium*, "of the womb"). Under the influence of hormones during each menstrual cycle, the cells that make up this layer get messages and stimulation to divide and thicken the wall, just in case there is a fertilized egg to cushion. When fertilization doesn't occur, the lining of the uterus gets the message to slough off and start thickening for the next cycle. The layer of cells and blood sloughed off each month constitute menstrual bleeding.

Endometriosis is a condition in which the endometrial cells, which belong only inside the uterus, show up in other places—on ovaries, bowel, bladder, ligaments or other structures in the abdominal cavity, or remote places such as lungs and even nasal mucosa. This condition might begin with one endometrial cell that acts as though it is in the uterine lining. It multiplies and divides each month. This cellular growth is stimulated by the normal cycle of sex hormones. But because this is happening outside of the uterus, there's no vaginal outlet for the thickened group of cells (menstrual blood).

Each month, the misplaced cells increase their numbers and slowly grow into a mass. This mass is benign (not cancerous), but still destructive. It causes scarring and a phenomenon known as *adhesions,* in which the sticky blood "glues" layers of tissues together. As the "glue" hardens, movement causes new rips and new sticky blood to worsen these adhesions. This partly explains why the dominant symptom of endometriosis is pain.

The unpredictable locations of uterine endometrial cells can cause symptoms as bizarre as nosebleeds or pink, frothy sputum with each menstrual cycle. Because these cells respond to menstrual hormones as the normal endometrial cells do, blood is trapped each month somewhere in the body. Old blood becomes oxidized and dark, giving the name "chocolate cyst" to encapsulated pockets of endometrial lesions. This highly toxic load causes cell destruction, intense pain, and a cascade of physical changes.

This allopathic definition is only half the answer for herbalists and others concerned with integrated medicine. It seems incomplete to accept the pathological description as the cause.

Symptoms and Signs

Common symptoms of endometriosis include cyclical pain, dysmenorrhea, and infertility. Lack of ovulation (anovulation) is associated with overgrowth of uterine endometrial tissue, while endometrial lesions on ovaries and fallopian tubes can block conception. Pain associated with menses frequently starts a week before bleeding and lasts for two to three days. Unlike the typical pain of dysmenorrhea (in which cramping is felt in the central abdomen), endometrial pain is often felt in the vagina, lower back, and lower abdomen. Scar tissue from endometrial lesions may attach to other structures; these can be painful when uterine spasms pull on uterine muscles or surrounding tissues.

Sharp stabbing pain comes and goes. Pelvic aching or burning sensations may not be limited to the time of menstruation. There may be pain at ovulation. There may be frequent or constant pain over the site of an endometrial lesion, yet there may be referred pain in distant sites, especially between the neck and shoulders. Pain that is relieved by ordinary treatment is a significant symptom of endometriosis. If you experience frequent back pain, nausea before every period, or pain with deep intercourse, a bowel movement, or urination, it is wise to get a diagnosis.

The pain associated with endometriosis may also interfere with sleep or cause depression or fatigue. Digestive symptoms include a swollen abdomen or intestinal gas. In more advanced cases, inflammation may lead to pinched nerve pain.

A pelvic examination may reveal tender nodules, or the ovaries may feel tender and enlarged. Diagnosis is usually confirmed by ultrasound (bouncing sound waves around inside to build up a picture) or laparoscopy (putting a periscope down into the pelvic basin and looking around).

The disease can develop slowly or be confused with other conditions. Endometriosis is suspected if pelvic pain is worsening without other explanation, or if a woman with premenstrual syndrome is not responding to one's best holistic atten-tion (see Chapter 4: PMS).

Cause

How does it happen that the right cell gets in the wrong place? The cause is not un-derstood by conventional Western medicine. However, several risk factors have been noted in many women with endometriosis:

- estrogen excess
- progesterone deficiency
- magnesium deficiency
- essential fatty acid deficiency (diet low in fresh seeds, nuts, grains)
- high-fat diet, especially animal fats (meat, dairy)
- high stress load, often complicated by hypoglycemia (low blood sugar)
- hormone imbalance
- excess dietary caffeine
- excess alcohol

Other predisposing factors include previous surgeries or interventions in tissue integrity—any surgery in which the uterine lining is touched by surgical instru-ments. A hereditary pattern is suggested by the fact that sisters are six times more likely to develop endometriosis than are their brothers' female partners.

The most consistent risk factor is severe stress, especially of a sexual nature. This could be a physical stress, such as having a Cesarean section or an ill-fitting IUD, or it could be a combination of physical and emotional distress. The sexual stress may be external, such as abusive relationships ranging from low-grade chronic domestic problems to rape. Stress may also be internal; for example when a distorted self-image leads to behavior changes and health degradation. And there may be nonsexual stress, ranging from living with environmental degradation to job or family pressures.

There is a strong suggestion that endometriosis is more than just the right cell in the wrong place. It has to do with relationship, both physical and nonphysical. The problem may be a stressful or "wrong" love relationship, or it may be too close a "relationship" with a toxic dump, paper mill, or nuclear power plant.

New information links dioxin from industrial bleaching with endometriosis. We are exposed to dioxin in our diet. Since dioxin is fat-soluble, it is concentrated in beef, milk, chicken, pork, fish, and eggs. Women also absorb dioxin from commer-cial tampons.

A 1992 study done in Germany showed that endometriosis is also correlated with PCBs (polychlorinated biphenyls—toxic industrial chemicals) from the environment found in humans.[1] PCBs and dioxin both interfere with the immune system and the endocrine system (the body's chemical control system made up of endocrine glands, which produce hormones).

Researchers have suspected for some time that endometriosis is somehow caused by malfunction of both the immune and endocrine systems. Dioxin and PCBs are not the only potential culprits. As Dr. Theo Colborn has shown, at least forty-five chemicals widely distributed in the environment, including thirty-five pesticides and one industrial chemical, are now thought to damage or impair the endocrine systems of fish, birds, and mammals, including humans.[2]

Unpredictable mutations, unexplainable female pathology—biological warfare isn't just in Vietnam or the Persian Gulf. One cannot claim that dioxin or even nuclear energy causes endometriosis; the industries that produce these and other "endodisruptors" generate well-funded studies to deny the evidence. Certainly nobody has studied the many unwieldy potential cofactors. There is no profit in such research, and the methodology would be intimidating to any serious team of researchers.

This epidemic of reproductive malfunction is probably not due simply to improved techniques of diagnosis, as has been claimed by medical personnel in the past. In previous decades, the formerly rare disease of endometriosis was presumed by a medical profession to occur among women who somehow brought it on themselves: older women without children (supposedly a frustrated maternal urge), "loose" women who had multiple surgeries (D&Cs, abortions, other procedures) or STDs (sexually transmitted diseases).

But now endometriosis occurs in all kinds of women, including healthy eighteen-year-old girls with no history of a serious reproductive infection or abortion. Endometriosis is most common among women between the ages of twenty and forty, and may subside after menopause.

Other possible causes of endometriosis have been theorized:

• The transportation theory: Reflux or retrograde menstrual flow, during uterine spasms of menstruation or severe dysmenorrhea, causes cells shed in menstruation to spurt from the fallopian tubes out into the abdominal cavity. Behind the *transportation theory* is the idea that living endometrial cells in the menstrual material

1. I. Gerhard und B. Runnebaum, *Grenzen der Hormonsubstitution bei Schadstoffbelastung und Fertilitatsstorungen,* "Zentralblatt fur Gynakologie," Vol. 114 (1992), pp. 593–602.

2. Theo Colborn, et al., "Developmental Effects of Endocrine-Disrupting Chemicals in Wildlife and Humans," *Environmental Health Perspectives,* Vol. 101 No. 5 (October 1993), pp. 378–384.

can implant on ovaries, bowel, bladder, or other structures within the pelvis, including the peritoneum that lines the pelvic basin. This does not explain why not all menstruating women get endometriosis.

- The formation in situ theory: Hormonal changes or aggravated inflammation may trigger abnormal cell changes, possibly turning other types of epithelial cells (covering a surface, organ, or tissue) into endometrial epithelial cells. Wherever this happens the endometrial cells respond to the next cycle of circulating hormones in the blood, especially estrogen, which stimulates their division into a cluster.

- The induction theory (mixture of the transportation and the formation in situ theories): The endometrial lining may induce other types of cells from deeper tissue layers to become endometrial epithelium.

- The embolic theory: The lymphatic vessels and veins surrounding the uterus may carry viable (living) endometrial cells shed during menses to distant sites. This is considered less likely than other causes.

- The congenital theory: A woman's endometrial cells were misplaced while she was still an embryo. These would become active endometrial cells during the hormonal trigger of puberty or later in reproductive life, so their presence in places other than the uterus would cause no symptoms until then. Though there is a strong hereditary pattern with endometriosis, congenital abnormalities of many kinds have been traced to environmental influences upon the pregnant mother.

Conventional Medical Care

If a woman is still fertile (endometriosis can decrease fertility through scarring), pregnancy and prolonged breast-feeding can give her a respite from endometriosis. This helps the body self-repair because the longer the woman goes without a menstrual period, the greater the hope of the condition being self-limiting.

Hormone drugs are used to treat endometriosis, including high-dose forms of progesterone, the birth control pill, Danazol, Lupron, Depo-Provera, and Norplant. These are considered ineffective or at least problematic on more than one count. They may lessen inflammation but not necessarily endometriosis, and some hormone drugs even allow pregnancy.

Danazol is a male hormone drug that works by reducing FSH and LH levels and costs a dollar per dose; it is taken for six to nine months at a time. Women who use it may experience side effects including pseudomenopause, hot flashes, a dry vagina, joint pain, weight gain, depression, irritability, fatigue, and voice changes. In extreme cases, side effects may include masculinization. There is a high rate of recurrent pain after pregnancy for those who conceive after this treatment. In addition, over 30% of these women have some kind of problem with fertility later on.

Common treatments such as Lupron (a monthly injection), Zolarex (a monthly implant), and Synarel (a nasal spray) are not cures; one of their effects is to lower estrogen levels until the woman reaches menopause.

The other main treatment prescribed by the medical establishment is removal of the endometrial lesions, which often fails even when the whole uterus is removed because the lesions are rarely limited to that organ.

Herbal Treatment

Holistic herbal treatments have been at least as helpful as surgery and hormonal drugs, except in medical emergencies. Because of the lack of clarity regarding the cause and nature of endometriosis, natural therapists keep an open mind for new understanding about effective treatment. Meanwhile, we can agree that endometriosis is a multifactorial condition. Varying degrees of success have been obtained by treating as many of the known cofactors as possible.

Herbs seem to promote tissue healing through a blend of effects. In addition to using phytoestrogens and other hormone-balancing plants, therapy aims to augment circulation to and from the areas of damage. Nutritive herbs provide building materials for the cells. Particular hepatic herbs may be chosen if a woman needs to eliminate toxins. Finally, it is important to improving immune-system function so that white blood cells will cluster around and eat up debris or imperfect cells.

Some women choose to forego any diagnostic microsurgery, on the theory that it may cause the very condition being identified. These women decide to undergo natural treatment for endometriosis without the certainty of a medical diagnosis. They reason that if the signs and symptoms respond successfully, the herbal "prescription" was correct for the presumed diagnosis.

My strong preference is for such a welcome disappearance of symptoms to be verified by follow-up with a licensed health care provider. This helps ensure a genuine return to wholeness and sustainable, vibrant health.

But how can we use herbs to correct the problem of healthy cells in the wrong place? Starting with adaptogen and analgesic herbs for the pain of physical, emotional, or psycho-spiritual distress allows women to draw a deep breath and think more clearly about longer-term management. Judgments about a woman's past medical history or her bad attitude toward herself, or even rationalizations about her "bad karma" are not useful.

To attend to the woman with this pathology we must delve deeper than conventional concepts, yet we cannot ignore them. The more we understand about the body, the more we can understand how our herbs can effectively support what is healthy. Knowing the site of endometrial lesions can help a woman choose an herb to normalize cellular integrity for that type of tissue, from nose to toes. But we are still left with the limitation that herbs only promote natural functions. The endometrial cell is in fact functioning as it normally does. Do herbs attack normal tissues that are causing disease by being in the wrong place? Not exactly, but if immunity is given optimal support, it has the programming to destroy disordered tissues that are "lost" or causing trouble. The herbs in the following formulas seem to work by combining cleansing effects with hormone-balancing properties and nonspecific support for immune-system regulation.

Although there is no magic cure, herbal treatment, improved nutrition, and visualization have helped women with diagnosed endometriosis to postpone or avoid surgery. This has sometimes happened with the blessing of their bewildered medical doctors. Sometimes women haven't told their physicians they were taking herbs. They just smiled mysteriously when the physicians canceled surgery, recommending no further treatment.

In herbal treatment, our objective is to restore the integrity of the uterine lining. In part, this is done by increasing the body's ability to deconstruct and scavenge inappropriately placed tissue. It seems that we do this by regulating hormonal balance and clearing obstruction, though we frankly admit that our perceived mechanism is uncertain. Nevertheless, the human results encourage cautious confidence.

The most narrow context of herbal treatment is aimed at reducing excess estrogen and increasing progesterone levels, with immune support, nervous system tonics, antispasmodics, and antimicrobials to prevent secondary infection in a stagnated system. In a wider view, women may need all the relevant physiological methods of promoting self-healing.

The following herbs, which will help most women, are given as two formulas for the two halves of the menstrual cycle. As with all formulas in this book, these formulas can be made milder or stronger, or customized to simultaneously help correct a secondary health imbalance.

There are several areas for women to consider before changing the formulas below to suit their own needs:

• Herbal Hepatics and the Liver: These herbs focus on hormone metabolism, improving the bile–bowel functional relationship, and treating gastrointestinal toxicity, flora, and pelvic blockage. Choose from *Rosmarinus* (rosemary leaves and flowers), *Taraxacum* (dandelion root and leaf), *Carduus marianum* (milk thistle seeds), and *Verbena officinalis* (vervain herb). Other hepatics, cholagogues, and alteratives may replace any one of these, according to the bioregional flora (what grows near you in abundance), the other actions, and the relevance to each particular woman.

• Cleansing: There may be a need for elimination beyond reliance on the hepatics listed above. This includes fasts alternating with rebuilding diets containing kelp, seaweed, sprouted seeds, and easily digested whole foods to speed recovery. Non-standard means of elimination should not be scorned, as the humble castor oil pack is effective in assisting recovery when placed over adhesions or the site of greatest pain (see Chapter 2: Herbal Preparation).

• Anti-inflammatories and Nervines: The primary symptom of pain impedes healing and must be treated with effective herbal nervines and analgesics while the more comprehensive state of health is slowly improving. The anti-inflammatory herb *Matricaria recutita* (chamomile flower) is useful here. Muscle relaxants such as the *Viburnum spp.* (cramp bark), *Valeriana* (valerian root) and *Humulus* (hops flower) are effective, though *Humulus* has a cold quality in common with other bitters. The heat-producing *Zingiber officinalis* (ginger root) relaxes muscles. The dried herb of *Anemone pulsatilla* (pasque flower herb) prepared as a tea, capsule, or tincture is a standard remedy in European phytotherapy (plant therapy) for reproductive pain and infection; herbalists in the United States report no ill effects from using fresh extracts.

• Lymphatic Circulation: This will assist delivery of the other herbs to improve the blood and lymph drainage. *Galium aparine* (cleavers), *Calendula* (calendula flower), and *Echinacea spp.* (purple coneflower root, seed) all work against a possible secondary infection due to stasis (stagnation), and *Echinacea*'s effects on collagen repair in connective tissue adds to its alterative and immune-system normalizing functions.

• Tonic Diuretics: Elimination through the kidneys allows the body's mechanisms for self-regulation to work optimally, while preventing buildup of stimulating herbs. *Solidago virgaurea* (goldenrod herb tea) prevents overtaxing the kidneys.

• Digestive Aids: Two types, demulcents and bitters, act in their respective ways. Demulcents such as *Althaea officinalis* (marshmallow root) soothe inflammation and reduce pain by reducing stimuli to pain sensors in the digestive mucosa. This has a reflex soothing effect through spinal nerve pathways to muscles other than digestive structures, which may be in spasm. This cannot ever be strong enough to completely suppress the warning symptom of inflammation, but decreasing the pain has healing effects. Bitters such as *Verbena* (vervain) or *Achillea* (yarrow herb) change the intestinal flora, or tone the bowel wall while stimulating general digestive function.

• Skin Alteratives: *Smilax ornata* (sarsaparilla root) gives tone rather than stimulation of the immune system. It is considered by herbalists to be a tonic for lymphatic circulation and hormonal balance, with an affinity for clearing skin conditions. Also in this category are two stronger skin alteratives with an effect on immunity, *Larrea mexicana* (chaparral) and *Berberis aquifolium* (Oregon grape).

• Expectorants: Mildly expectorant diaphoretics may overlap with the benefits of alteratives by warming the circulation. Herbs chosen for strengthening elimination through the respiratory organs may have other benefits. British medical herbalist Sue Godwin writes that *Cimicifuga racemosa* (black cohosh) may play a role in dissolving adhesions while carrying out its better-known actions of clearing lungs, relaxing muscle, calming nerves, and normalizing reproductive cycles. Though Rudolph Weiss calls *Cimicifuga* an estrogenic plant, herbalists use it for its antispasmodic role in a protocol for endometriosis.

• Astringents: Both metrorrhagia (bleeding between periods) and internal bleeding (endometrial or from ruptures) are affected. Fresh plant tincture or preparation of *Capsella bursa-pastoris* (shepherd's purse) will decrease abnormal bleeding, as will *Hamamelis virginiana* (witch hazel bark), *Agrimonia eupatoria* (agrimony herb), *Hydrastis canadensis* (goldenseal root), and *Vinca spp.* (periwinkle herb). Since goldenseal is endangered and good quality agrimony is hard to find in many regions, fresh *Capsella bursa-pastoris* (shepherd's purse) tincture may be the best bet.

• Nervine Tonics: These reduce tension and take the edge off pain since the symptoms can be so difficult to manage. These synergize with analgesics and include *Leonurus cardiaca* (motherwort herb, also a bitter), *Scutellaria spp.* (skullcap herb), and flower essences. Flower essences are a gentle, practically etheric way of using the essences of plants in water. This is not the internal use of essential oils, but an energy imprint or vibration of a plant form, used to affect one's thoughts and emotional states.

Herbalists take natural advantage of the changes in each phase of a woman's menstrual cycle, using herbs to accentuate the desired direction of hormonal rebalancing. The purpose of the Herbal Formula I is to decrease excess estrogen during the luteal phase of the cycle. The purpose of Herbal Formula II is to balance progesterone and to shrink and heal endometrial lesions.

Plants in both formulas share complementary effects throughout the month; these relax painful spasms, stimulate liver function, build healthy immune-system response to cellular debris, or nourish a woman undergoing the physiological demands of self-healing.

Herbal formula I

(taken from ovulation through the end of menses)

Vitex agnus-castus (chasteberry seed)	1 ounce
Viburnum opulus (cramp bark)	2 ounces
Achillea millefolium (yarrow flower)	2 ounces
Scutellaria lateriflora (skullcap herb)	2 ounces
Dioscorea villosa (wild yam root)	1 ounce

Herbal Formula II

(taken from the end of menses to ovulation)

Vitex agnus-castus (chasteberry seed)	2 ounces
Caulophyllum thalictroides (blue cohosh root)	1 ounce
Smilax ornata (sarsaparilla root)	1 ounce
Carduus marianum (milk thistle seed)	2 ounces
Mitchella repens (partridgeberry herb)	1 ounce
Dioscorea villosa (wild yam root)	2 ounces

Optional:

Valeriana officinalis (valerian root)	1 ounce or more

If the pain is severe but you are sensitive to *Valeriana,* you may be replace it with double the amount or more of *Passiflora* (passionflower herb).

The directions and dosage for both of these formulas are standard; see Chapter 2: Herbal Preparation. These must be continued for a minimum of three months before effects may have a lasting benefit, but the therapy should improve symptoms of pain within the first few days. The complete treatment would take into account the length of the disease and its progression. An average length of one year is absolutely normal.

Taking herbs becomes a routine part of a woman's daily self-care, like brushing her teeth. Granted, it isn't as quick as surgery, but it allows us to get to the cause. Long-term herbal self-care also encourages healthy habits for life, and it only takes fifteen minutes every three days to make a big pitcher of tea or a few weeks of shaking a jar to make a year's worth of tincture.

Herbs can right the body's internal signals for tissue growth, relax taut muscles, calm the mind, and smooth a woman's emotional turmoil. But can just ingesting an herbal compound get to the cause behind these factors? Herbs play a supportive role in this discovery of self and relationship. The causative problems respond to a healthy balance of physical action (taking herbs, avoiding red meat) and meditation—personally, culturally, and globally.

External Treatments

Essential oils of geranium, cypress, and clary sage may be massaged over areas of discomfort. They can also be used as aromatherapy in the form of hand and foot baths, sitz baths (three drops total per bath), or steam inhalations and old-fashioned room vaporizers. This last form works especially well for softening barriers to self-knowledge with female sexuality and abuse issues.

Nutrition

Nutritional changes include avoiding caffeine, sugar, alcohol, and acid-forming foods (red meat, dairy products, heated or treated oils, and excess carbohydrates, especially refined products).

Try a short juice fast to clear out the body, and follow up with cultured foods such as miso or tempeh, unless you have a food allergy to soy products. After cleansing the body, plenty of fresh greens, fresh fruits in season, and a reasonable quantity of whole grains provide strength. Include changes to stabilize hypoglycemia (low blood sugar), such as eating smaller meals. As always, eating little or no animal fat decreases harmful excess estrogen. What meat you do eat should be raised organically.

Too many supplements can be hard for a body to digest, especially during illness. Please rely on local, high-quality food for most of your vitamins and minerals. Levels of vitamin B complex are high in grains and green leafy vegetables, molasses, and brewer's yeast.

Supplements

I recommend the following amounts daily:

vitamin B complex (containing 2 milligrams B_6): use as directed on label

folic acid: 150 micrograms

liquid potassium: taken in recommended doses, 3 times a day

flax seed oil: start at ⅛-teaspoon doses; increase to 1 teaspoon per dose or more as tolerated

vitamin E: 8–10 milligrams alpha-TE (alpha tocopherol equivalent); may use 200–600 IU (up to 1,200 IU maximum)

herb/vegetable iron supplement (available in natural food stores, or see Liquid "Maid of Iron" Formula in Chapter 7: Anemia).

magnesium: 400 milligrams

calcium: 800 milligrams

vitamin A: 800 RE (retinol equivalent); may use 5,000 IU (up to 50,000 IU for four months or less)

vitamin D: 10 RE; may use 400 IU (up to 1,000 IU maximum)

vitamin C: 300 milligrams (up to 10 grams)

evening primrose oil (for GLA—gamma-linolenic acid): eight 500-milligram capsules per day for six to ten weeks, if women can afford this dose (most effective)

Though there is good evidence suggesting that lower doses of evening primrose oil (EPO) are of value for reproductive imbalance (breast tenderness, PMS), my experience is that higher doses are more effective for reproductive damage (inflammation, pain). Other sources of essential fatty acids such as flax, borage, or black currant seed oil are important for a rounded intake of healthy oils, but these do not act as quickly in women with endometriosis. For this reason, I prefer to use higher doses of the more expensive EPO for the short term.

Exercise

Despite pain, women with endometriosis are encouraged to exercise gently in ways that move the pelvis and release tension. Walking or moving without gravity in water (heated pools, leg-kicks in large hot tubs) may be enough exertion for some women. Others may prefer to work out intensely. Be aware of your own tolerance for forceful or rapid movement, which may worsen adhesions. Endometriosis lesions can rupture, so pay attention to your body and be careful while gaining fitness.

Other Points

Even in minute amounts, X rays are thought by some alternative practitioners to potentiate (bring on or worsen) inappropriate or excessive tissue growth. Sonograms are slightly preferred, but these have their own drawbacks. Sonograms may be overused diagnostic tools, though physicians claim that the use of this technique saves lives by "reading" the structures that threaten a woman's life. These medical technologies should be viewed with reservation and are best avoided as a diagnostic tool, unless it is a matter of the utmost importance to bounce sound waves off sensitive tissues already presumed damaged. The effects are not proven safe beyond all question. Diagnosis for endometriosis usually relies not on sonogram readings, but on laparoscopy.

Don't use IUDs or tampons until you are healthy (showing no symptoms and in a positive state of health) for six consecutive months. Menstrual sea sponges are not great alternatives to tampons. My experience is that they crumble and cause infections, even when sterilized and dried between use as directed. Unbleached, nondeodorant cotton pads are safe. Natural food stores and herb shops carry washable flannel cloths for menstruation.

Join a local support group or take a women's awareness class to identify personal cofactors and realistic means for addressing them. National groups may be more medically conservative than I am, but they are well-informed about effective treatment women have experienced and sources for additional support:

The Endometriosis Alliance
P.O. Box 326
Cooper Station
New York, NY 10276-0326

The Endometriosis Association
8585 North 76th Place
Milwaukee, WI 53223
Fax: (414) 355-6065

Families affected by the disease can call the association's toll-free line (800-992-3636) for a free packet of information.

Relaxation, visualization, breathing exercises and counseling all have their value. Emotional clearing may be as simple as screaming in a safe place every once in a while or lying in the shade of a favorite tree.

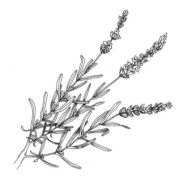

13

Fibrocystic Breast Tissue

BENIGN BREAST CYSTS

Definition

What exactly is fibrocystic breast disease? The "disease" is the development of benign breast lumps, from very small to very large (pinhead- to pea- to marble- or golf-ball-size). These lumps, which are far more common than breast cancer, are often misinterpreted by women and their doctors. They don't cause or predispose us to breast cancer.

Fibrocystic breast disease sounds awful, but most women above the age of twenty-four in the western hemisphere have it to some degree. Many women aren't aware of it until it is identified during a routine exam by a health care provider. This common condition responds well to gentle holistic methods, including nutritional changes, herbs, and external remedies.

Our breasts contain glands near the chest wall that can make milk when the hormones of pregnancy begin "activating" them. They respond to our hormonal changes every month; women who are not mothers and those who breast-feed are equally likely to have lumps, especially if there is significant stress, coffee, and some synthetic hormones.

Symptoms and Signs

Painful breasts are not natural, but they are common. Some premenstrual tenderness is normal, but pain is not healthy. What does it mean about the world we inhabit—or women's collective response to our world—that painful breasts are so normal these days?

The breasts are responding to triggers that may herald any number of other breakdowns in reproductive health. Herbalists prefer not to wait until the body comes up with a more serious disease before turning to preventive herbal care.

With benign breast lumps, there may be tenderness or even pain before periods or after gaining weight, or simply an unusual degree of tenderness after bumping into things. These simple cofactors of breast tenderness are frequently missed by physicians looking for pathology.

Often there are no painful symptoms other than the emotional concern caused by feeling lumps upon examining the breasts. Depending on the number of cysts present, breasts may have a few little "peas" under the skin that move around, or the breast may feel like a bag of lentils.

Cause

Our minds and hearts cause our endocrine glands to make hormones. A few of these in turn make our breasts swell, shrink, flow with milk, or dry up. Sometimes healthy breasts are still a little lumpy. This is especially true if we are drinking coffee, eating meat and dairy products, under stress, or relatively high in our estrogen levels.

It is important for each woman to know what her "normal lumps" of healthy breast tissue feel like so that she can self-monitor any new breast lumps. Guidance from an experienced health care professional helps rule out serious problems. In past years this noncancerous disease was said to predispose women to breast cancer, but that relationship has since been questioned. Even though they don't cause cancer, benign lumps may hide cancerous lumps. Many of the factors associated with benign breast lumps, such as hormonal imbalance, high stress, and low vitamin A, may in themselves "cooperate" in a breakdown of health that could progress to cancer.

In older texts, benign breast lumps are called "chronic cystic mastitis." The ending *-itis* means inflammation, but it isn't really like the mastitis of pregnancy or breast-feeding. Benign breast lumps are really a hyperplasia, or abnormal overgrowth of otherwise normal tissue.

Benign breast lumps occur anytime between puberty and menopause. New benign cysts do not usually appear after menopause unless a woman takes hormone replacement. Hormone replacement prolongs estrogen stimulation to the breast tissue and short-circuits the body's menopausal hormone shift—a time when fibrous overgrowths would otherwise tend to shrink.

There are several types of common benign breast lumps. Sometimes breast-feeding mothers have a blocked milk duct that ruptures and scars over, but it may be felt as a lump later. This is called *duct ectasia.*

Fat necrosis literally means dead fatty tissue. Relax; it's one of those terrific descriptions of what happens when an injury to breasts occurs, as with hockey players or horse riders. More disturbingly, such injury is common among battered women. Damaged structures may force emboli (a blood clot loose in the blood stream) to block a small blood vessel and possibly cause localized tissue "death." However, it is part of life that our immune system mops up such damage when immunity isn't overloaded or suppressed.

A type of benign lump that young women tend to have is a rubbery, round pea that can be moved around easily in the breast tissue during an examination. These are *fibroadenomas,* and they may or may not be removed. On rare occasion, one of these may grow quite large, rapidly, but it is still not malignant. They usually go away with age, as they are estrogen-dependent and only require conventional medical attention if there are other signs of worsening disease. If removed, these tend to grow back, but they rarely spread to lymph nodes. Regrowth is a signal to the woman that underlying causes have not been altered: choice of food, habits, environment.

Sometimes recurring breast changes signal us that we're still under an effect that we can't change. These may be as uncertain as heredity, DES given to our mothers, or any of the following factors reported by women investigating the roots of their disease: heavy-gauge power lines nearby; radiation from television, computer screens, and microwaves; or a combination of small negative health risks from an unholy smorgasbord of environmental horrors.

Benign lumps usually occur in both breasts, but they may be unequally distributed, or there may be only one or two cysts. What happens is that normal structures for milk production get overstimulated, swollen, and filled in. The milk ducts dilate into little cysts or sacs that may fill with fluid. After a while, the tissue returns to normal unless the overstimulation continues.

If overstimulation does continue, the body makes what it considers a reasonable decision to turn the fluid into a semisolid gel that is part water, part fat, part mucus, and part fibrous tissue. Some version of this process of "patching and repair" is how our body tries to heal any group of stressed, inflamed, swollen, or unstable cells. After a while, fibrous tissue fills the sacs solid. At this point, we may feel lumps. Every month during the menstrual cycle, the upsurge in estrogen and the change of other hormones triggers activity, new swelling, and a little more pressure backing up around these solidifying ducts.

Up to a certain point this process is reversible, but it takes time. Think of the thick, white scars on new wounds; over time they are replaced by normal skin cells. Similarly, reversing cystic changes in breast tissue relies on removal of stimulants to breast tissue as well as taking herbs that are focused on lymph drainage and a state of "neuroendocrine calm."

Our breasts are objects of much importance to our infants and to our evolving self-image, from prepuberty into old age. Western culture does not yet teach women that their mammary glands belong to them. Breasts are still treated as commodities, central to the industry driven by male fantasy, which makes our breasts worth millions of dollars annually in car sales or ads for liquor. Rarely do a woman's breasts earn *her* millions of dollars a year.

Conventional Medical Care

From the conventional medical viewpoint, treatment is rarely required. Persistent pain, changes to breast skin, or other signs a woman is at high risk require follow-up. Your health care provider can determine what treatment might be indicated.

Herbal Treatment

The herbs that can slow, stop, or reverse formation of lumps in the breast do so by increasing lymph vessel circulation in the breast tissue while optimizing hormonal balance. These herbs include *Smilax ornata* (sarsaparilla root) and *Vitex agnus-castus* (chasteberry). (For others, see "Hormonal Tonics" in Chapter 1: Herbal Glossary).

Herbs that help women alter stress patterns will also reduce overstimulation of sensitive tissue. These are the nervine relaxants, such as *Verbena officinalis* (vervain herb). Altering stress patterns includes easing the stress of crummy food choices on the body. Bitter herbs and adaptogens keep our appetites on track to avoid sugar cravings or nervous eating.

The herbs in the following formulas are too gentle to override a woman's mindset, but powerful enough to anchor her hope for restoring healthier breast tissue.

Herbal Formulas

This three-part formula gives women a rich, earthy cup of root tea and two blossom-filled cups of fairy light every day, plus a single concentrated plant extract (tincture) to act as a bridge between matter and spirit.

Herbal Formula, Part I

Arctium lappa (burdock root)	5 ounces
Carduus marianum (milk thistle seed)	4 ounces
Phytolacca decandra (poke root)	1 ounce
Smilax ornata (sarsaparilla root)	3 ounces

Oplopanax horridum (devil's club)	1 ounce
Vitex agnus-castus (chasteberry seed)	2 ounces

Decoct (simmer) 1 ounce of herbs in 3 cups of water for fifteen minutes on medium-low heat; strain and drink 1 cup daily. Tea will last three days in refrigerator. Sixteen ounces of herb mixture will last for over six weeks at this dose. Continue for a minimum of three months.

Herbal Formula, Part II

Calendula officinalis (calendula flower)	1 ounce
Viola odorata (sweet violet leaf and flower)	1 ounce
Melissa officinalis (lemon balm leaf and flower)	1 ounce
Verbena officinalis (vervain leaf)	1 ounce
Lippia citriodora (lemon verbena leaf and flower)	3 ounces

Infuse (steep) one tablespoon of herbal mixture in a pint of water for fifteen minutes; strain and drink 2 cups daily for three months.

Herbal Formula, Part III: Extract

Take one teaspoon of *Galium aparine* (cleavers herb—fresh, not dried) diluted in one eight-ounce glass of water or one cup of flower-herb tea, twice a day for three months. You may use a purchased extract or tincture if the label says that it is made from *fresh* plant material. Or make your own *Galium* extract by following the instructions on making tinctures in Chapter 2: Herbal Preparation. Plan this little job for the spring or early summer, when cleavers is in season. Ask any organic farmer, gardener, or local botanical group to show you fresh cleavers. Cleavers is like gold to herbalists, but a pesky "weed" to others, and can be found in most growing zones of North America and Europe, with the exception of most of the southwestern deserts.

External Herbal Therapies

Choose the external therapy that appeals to you most and that you will be reasonably consistent in doing. The variety of external herbal recipes offered here is not intended to confuse you, but to give you a choice. All of these have worked, yet all of them have failed for some woman somewhere sometime. Experiment to find the one that works for you.

Continue using one until any drainage stops, breast lumps are gone, or one to three months of consistent efforts have gone by. Applying herbs externally once a week helps a little; four to five times a week may show results in two to four weeks. If an external treatment brings you little improvement within this time, try another method.

1. Take a towel soaked in hot water, and squeeze it out. Apply it hot over the affected area for three to five minutes to stimulate circulation.

Afterward, a compress may be applied over the area to help facilitate the discharge of accumulated matter. Take 2 ounces of any one or more of the following: green clay, kaolin clay, or bentonite clay; mix with 4 ounces of pounded-up cabbage leaves. A little water may be added to the mixture if it is too dry.

Good-quality clay can usually be obtained from a pottery studio or school teacher who uses fine clay. Alternatively, naturally colored clays (green, blue, rose) may be found in the cosmetic section of a natural food store.

Apply the mixture to the affected area; leave it in place and keep it moist and medium-warm for two hours. Use hot water bottles, occasionally refilled, and dry bath towels or blankets wrapped around the torso to keep things in place and warm. There is no harm in leaving it on overnight.

Ideally, do this in the evenings while sitting still, reading, dreaming or otherwise relaxing, every day for one month. If this is too much to do nightly, try it twice a week for up to three months.

It is worth the hassle. This compress gradually removes the excess mucus and fats from tissues. We do not know for sure how it works. Folklore says that the sticky mucus is drawn by the cabbage–clay mixture toward the surface of the skin. Eventually, lumps decrease in size. Some women report that they see the fatty mucus or sticky substances in the herb compress when it is removed. I cannot say I have ever seen this, though I have seen changes to softer breast tissue with smaller and fewer lumps. In any case, clay and cabbage are nontoxic.

2. A ginger compress can stimulate circulation of blood and body fluids. It helps loosen and dissolve stagnated toxic matter, and reduces the size of cysts and growths.

To prepare it, place a handful of grated fresh ginger root in a cheesecloth and squeeze out the ginger juice into one gallon of very hot water. Do not boil the water, or you will lose the volatile power (the essential oil you can smell in the fleshy root) of the ginger. Dip a cotton hand towel into the ginger water, wring it out tightly, and apply it, very hot but not uncomfortably so, to the whole area surrounding the lump. Cover the whole breast if it's easier. A second, dry towel can be placed on top to reduce heat loss.

Apply a fresh hot towel dipped in the ginger water every five minutes or as the cloth cools. Repeat until the skin becomes red. This can be done daily for up to one month before evaluating progress.

3. For a description of the castor oil compress, see Chapter 2: Herbal Preparation.

4. The classic poke compress is simple: put one-fourth to one-half ounce of warm tincture of poke root on a hand towel or piece of flannel; place this over the breast area for four hours or overnight.

Alternatively, a strong decoction (two ounces of dried poke root in eight ounces of simmering water for fifteen minutes) makes a fine poultice. Use the warm pulp and tea together to make a paste like thick, warm gravy. Apply it directly to the skin for twenty minutes, covered with a clean dry cloth and a hot water bottle to keep in heat. This opens skin pores and allows the herbal constituents to affect the breast through surface blood vessels.

If fresh grated poke root is available (ask an herb gardener), use one-half to one ounce with sufficient hot water to make a poultice. See Chapter 2: Herbal Preparation for more information if required.

Use any one or more of these forms of poke root compress nightly for up to one month before reevaluation.

Nutrition

Eliminate all caffeine-containing products: coffee (including decaffeinated or instant), chocolate and cocoa, black tea, colas, and other sodas. These all contain methylxanthines, a group of alkaloids that block the enzyme *phosphodiesterase*. When that happens, there is more formation of fibrous tissue, increased cell growth, and more fluid filling any existing cysts.

Eliminate hops as an herb or in beer. The plant may promote estrogen in women already sensitive to estrogenic stimulation, though this is not certain. As for the beer, alcohol combined with the plant sterols stimulates unhealthy activity of breast cells.

Reduce intake of dairy products, refined foods, and excess carbohydrates. These promote excess mucus and fat, which block decongesting herbs. Excess carbohydrates that our body can't burn as fuel get turned into fat for storage. Fat stores make estrogen. Fibrocystic breasts are your body's way of saying that you haven't metabolized existing loads of estrogen very well. Balancing your hormones means maintaining a healthy body weight.

Supplements

Daily recommendations include:

vitamin A: 25,000 IU for three weeks only; then drop the dose to 15,000 IU for another two weeks; then take 10,000 IU for two weeks; finally, follow with foods rich in beta-carotene and vitamin A

vitamin E: 600 to 1,000 IU (in severe hypertension, kidney disease, or diabetes mellitus, limit the dose to 200 IU daily)

Other Points

Exercises for the upper chest are recommended, fifteen to twenty minutes daily. Let it be fun as well as good for your health. Stretching, weights, aerobics, all kinds of dance from around the world, yoga, and even stationary breathing exercises are all good ways to bring circulation, oxygen, and free-flowing energy through the upper torso. The herbs won't get there if they can't circulate well in the bloodstream. And healthy veins are able to help the cells eliminate waste products every day.

If a woman with fibrocystic breasts is on the birth control pill, alternative contraception is recommended. The cervical cap is one option. Some women are satisfied with the natural method of birth control. This low-technology method relies on a woman charting basal metabolic temperature and cervical mucus. More reliable than the notorious rhythm method, the cooperative nature of this system involves male partners and requires them to be as responsible as women. This brings a sweet intimacy to the relationship over time. The natural method isn't great for one-night stands, but that kind of Russian roulette isn't a healthy sexual signal to give to one's vagina and uterus anyway.

Breasts are potent symbols of our womanhood. Venus, the archetype we know as the goddess of love, loves herself. She is a positive figure who exudes sensuality and a love of life. Venus is every woman when she isn't worn down or worried.

Women with a burden "on their chests" or fear in their breasts have so many pressing needs. Most women facing health issues in the twenty-first century perceive themselves as existing in a survival mode. Women in survival mode need beauty, not guilt; questions, not lectures.

Has your culture helped you love your breasts—or yourself, just the way you are? Does your love of self allow you to truly love others? If not, how would you change things?

To the extent that she has faith in herself, every woman has within her the power to recreate her world. If taking on a whole culture makes you feel like going back to bed for the rest of the day, just relax. Your contribution to the revolution is to go where you are loved. Unplug the television and watch an animal, even an ant. Go for a walk in a park. Find one healthy way to leave a crass culture behind; it has not loved you very truly anyway. What does this have to do with herbs for lumpy breasts? Everything.

Breast Self-Examination

The purpose of examining your own breasts is to get comfortable with your hands feeling your own normal lumps and bumps. Do this once a month at the same time each month, usually after menstruation if you are still having a reproductive cycle.

Position yourself in front of a mirror with good light. Let your arms drop naturally to your sides. Simply look. Notice the contour and color of breasts and nipples, especially discharge; some difference between breasts is normal. Repeat with your arms raised above your head, then place hands on hips while you contract your chest muscles.

Feel your breasts while lying down. Use your left hand to feel your right breast, then your right hand to feel your left. Place the arm you are not using with your hand resting comfortably up by your head. If you have small breasts (cup size A), fold a towel or place a small pillow under your back on the side you are feeling. If you have large breasts, lie on your back with your hips turned in the opposite direction of the breast you are examining.

The breast tissue is more than the mound that fits in a bra. Feel the edges of your breast from the collarbone to the first rib, from the center of the sternum (breastbone) to the armpit. Be sure to examine the whole armpit. Use the pads of three or four fingers together. Move fingers in small circles the size of a dime.

Since tumors may occur at any level, start by feeling the surface of the breast. Then repeat by feeling the middle layer, finally repeating with flats of fingers (pads, not pointing straight down) at the chest wall. Don't mistake your ribs for hard lumps attached to the muscle wall!

There are three major patterns to feel all of your breast:

1. Up and down strips: Move from the center of the body (ribs to collarbone) out to the armpit, using small circular movements (dime size) with pads of fingers.

2. Wedges of pie: Imagine your breast is a pie, or if you prefer, a wheel divided by 12 spokes. Examine each segment separately, using small circular motions from the outside to the nipple. Move your fingers out to the edge at the end of a segment, slide over a finger's width and examine the next section.

3. Spirals: Start at the center of the collarbone and move in a clockwise direction, slowly circling in with one long spiral with ever-smaller circles reaching the nipple.

Gently squeeze each nipple to check whether there is discharge. Small amounts of clear or white discharge may be normal for some women during the follicular (first half) of the menstrual cycle. If you have questions about your discharge, see your health care provider.

The first time a woman examines her breasts this thoroughly she will naturally have questions. It may take some time before each month's exam gives you confidence in your skill. Ask a midwife, nurse-practitioner, or your physician to watch how you examine your breasts. This is their job—to give feedback and guidance, explaining what you are feeling under your fingers. They cannot do this for you every month because self-exam is a major key to early detection and self-awareness. For many exams your breasts may feel the same. If there should be a change, ask your health care provider to help you interpret it.

PART FOUR

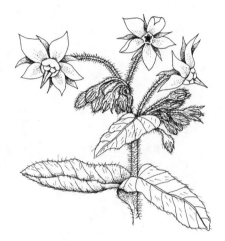

Healthy Reproduction

14

Clearing Blocks to Reproduction
INFERTILITY

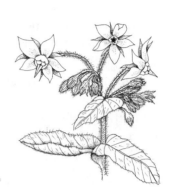

Definition

Infertility is defined both as difficulty in getting pregnant, and difficulty in maintaining a pregnancy to term. In this chapter, I will discuss herbs to help conception take place.

Infertility is not a problem with one partner or the other, no matter what the tests say. When a couple wants to conceive, any "failure" is of the unit, not either individual. Having a baby is simple, yet when it does not seem simple, it carries the complex baggage of culture.

Symptoms and Signs

In women who cannot conceive, there are signs that indicate whether and when the ovaries are working. A predictable change in temperature occurs immediately after ovulation. Changes can be tracked by taking daily readings of basal metabolic temperature (BMT). Basal body thermometers come with sample charts and instructions, and can be obtained from any good women's clinic or drugstore. This self-charting gives women exact days for trying to conceive (or to avoid conception).

This method is backed up by charting cervical mucus changes. Brief, clear notes on a daily chart allow a woman to "chart" her fertile cycle. Check well-stocked bookstores for books on natural fertility awareness.

Cause

Complex hormonal triggers are an internal conversation. Hormones have "voices" that carry messages from the hypothalamus to the pituitary in the brain. The pituitary is where FSH (follicle-stimulating hormone) is made. This hormone requests that the ovary allow one of its egg follicles to mature under this stimulating hormone's influence. The ovary, in turn, tells the hypothalamus how estrogen production, egg development, and indirectly, how the uterus lining is processing through changing levels of estrogen.

Too low or too high a level of any one of these hormones at any stage can cause or infertility. Infections may cause this, or a low thyroid function (hypothyroidism) may be a cause.

Causes of infertility include:

- age (over 40, especially for first pregnancy)
- allergies
- antibody production (to sperm or fetus)
- birth control pill use for several years in the past
- disease of either partner
- eggs not being released, perhaps due to imbalance of FSH
- exposure to chemicals, radiation, power lines, computers, electric blankets, or microwaves; digital clocks or LCDs (liquid crystal displays) near bed
- extremes of body weight
- low sperm count
- mucus of vaginal secretions hostile to sperm
- nutritional disturbances
- reproductive conditions: endometriosis, fibroids, PID, infections
- strenuous physical activity
- stress
- tilted uterus
- tough coating around eggs (barrier to sperm penetration)

A common cause of infertility that is often overlooked is a woman's weight. Sometimes simply gaining five or ten pounds changes her hormone levels enough to allow conception. On the other hand, some women carrying more than ten to twenty percent excess body fat may have problems conceiving because of the type of estrogen our body fat makes. Losing fifteen to twenty pounds may do more than allow a woman to conceive; when changes that accompany pregnancy make demands on her body, she will be better able to cope.

There are anatomic causes of infertility. One major cause is ovarian age. With age, our ovaries may release eggs too infrequently.

"Ovarian failure" is a clinically judgmental way of stating the obvious—that the ovaries are not releasing any mature, healthy eggs—but this does not explain why. Several reasons may explain ovarian failure, from birth defects to premature menopause. In some cases, all we may know for sure is that a woman experiences fewer or no menstrual cycles.

Menstrual bleeding is hormonally triggered when no fertilization occurs, so even without ovulation we know something is working if a woman is having menstrual bleeding more or less regularly.

Without periods at all, ovarian failure could be due to many things. A common reason is an insufficient numbers of eggs, or eggs that are no longer viable. In ovarian failure, there is not enough hormonal input to adequately build up the lining of the womb, trigger ovulation, or trigger the following stage of menstrual bleeding. Unlike infertility due to simple hormone imbalance, in this case hormonal voices are silent due to the lack of a healthy egg as a starting point.

Other anatomic problem is scar tissue. Old scars from surgery or trauma might block fertilized eggs from implanting successfully in a uterine lining that is ready and waiting each month. Scar tissue formation after chronic infections such as PID (pelvic inflammatory disease) and endometriosis may cause infertility in this way. Ongoing damage from disease processes might cause infertility; it doesn't have to be an old problem in the past. Anatomical blocks in the fallopian tubes include scarring, being tied off, or surgical removal. This keeps sperm and egg from meeting. Local structural blockages such as severe scar tissue in the tubes require different techniques than herbal therapy. Castor oil packs (described in Chapter 2: Herbal Preparation) applied over areas of internal scarring may bring a change, though it may not be possible in all cases.

Other factors that create an environment unfavorable to sperm and egg include an IUD (intrauterine device), thick mucus plugs the body may pump out in response to chronic inflammation (IUD, infection), or a poor diet.

Healthy vaginal fluid is supposed to be slightly acidic. Nutrition or other factors may cause an alkaline pH that makes squiggly sperm go all limp and sleepy. Alkaline vaginal pH is traced to excess dietary sugar, starches, and alcohol.

Infections of reproductive tissues, including infections caused by IUDs, may be the cause as well as the result of vaginal pH problems. Antimicrobial herbs that can help resolve common infections are covered in Part 5. Infections must receive primary attention before pursuing fertility. Meanwhile, a change to a healthier diet always helps infections clear up as well as promoting fertility.

Another possible anatomical problem is that the cervix may produce a sticky mucus that traps sperm. Sperm prefer to swim like wild salmon up their favorite rivers for spawning in a slippery, smooth waterway of thin, fertile mucus mixed with alkaline secretions from semen.

Structural problems, especially from car accidents or sports injuries, may lead to a slight or exaggerated tightness in the pelvis. Structural blockages to nerve impulse, blood flow, and function may be lessened through massage, chiropractic care, osteopathy, and most importantly, exercise suited to the individual.

Stress levels are significant to hormonal balance and infertility. Infertility causes stress, and stress causes infertility. When women are infertile due to stress, they may not be making LH (luteinizing hormone). Low or no LH means that we stop ovulating, perhaps because our physical, mental, and emotional being senses that the stress affecting our blood and brain chemistry will not favor pregnancy at that time. Male infertility also requires consideration. It is a mystery of nature's abundance that countless sperm are required for the right chemical environment to allow that one sperm to enter and fertilize the egg. This may be just a survival mechanism, allowing the most active sperm to be the first to fertilize the healthy but passive egg. A less Darwinian view is that the numbers of other sperm assure that the seed of the father came from healthy, rich abundance, usually a good indicator of health.

Today, many males have low sperm counts. This may be part of the fertility issue women face today, since the normal range is lower these days than it has ever been since sperm counts have been recorded. The pattern of low sperm count increasing through the last century is due to factors that include environmental pollution, radiation, and other endocrine disruptors.

Conventional Medical Care

Tests done to measure infertility include: temperature (BMT), thickening of the endometrial lining, progesterone levels (indicating how well the ovarian follicles are producing this hormone), tests for immune antibodies, postcoital tests close to mid-cycle ovulation for cervical mucus assessment, injecting dye to X ray the structures for blockage, and direct inspection by laparoscopy (cutting through tissue layers for a look). Laparoscopy is somewhat like putting a periscope down through the belly button to get a good look around. It may turn up diagnostic information, but it is an assault to reproductive tissues presumably damaged enough to prevent fertility.

The conventional treatment is to give the missing hormone. This may cause secondary problems, which can be fixed with more hormones, such as administration of estrogen. Surgery may correct blockages, but it doesn't always. Endometriosis is treated with a synthetic drug to trick the body into thinking it is pregnant so it won't menstruate while on birth control pills, after surgical removal of lesions, or both.

At great emotional and financial cost, there are drugs that force a woman's body to mature and release eggs. Fertility drugs are the main reason there are so many twins, triplets, and other multiple births in recent years, especially in women who were previously unable to develop one viable egg.

Artificial insemination (AI, or in-vitro fertilization) also requires extra medication and an annoying frequency of tests. Statistics on success rates may be misleadingly optimistic, and this approach is guaranteed to be more consuming of time and money than anyone expects at the outset.

Frozen embryos seem a workable but symbolically difficult way to start one's life.

Surrogate motherhood is clearly gambling with the hearts of more than the parents, and can hardly be recommended as a healing proposition anymore. It never ends as the people involved intended when they set out.

Herbal Treatment

The holistic objective is to promote health, including optimum weight and reproductive function in both partners. Natural fertility treatment for one adult partner takes the other's support and participation into account whenever that would be helpful to their shared goal of having a healthy baby. It doesn't hurt for a man to make a woman's daily tea or to drink a cup of raspberry leaf tea with her. And I provide an herbal formula in this section for men to use when tests indicate their health can be improved in an integrated approach to fertility.

Knowing the cause of infertility in each couple's case is necessary for treatment. Yet, no matter what the cause, treatment is more likely to succeed if the couple agrees to avoid polarizing on "her flaw," "his problem," "my genes," "your job."

In some cases of infertility, a woman's immune-system cells consider the sperm cells foreign protein to be attacked; medicinal plants to normalize immune-system function can then be used.

Both partners might also spend a few months before conception taking alterative immunomodulators such as *Lentinus edodes* (shiitake mushrooms), *Ganoderma spp.* (reishi mushrooms), or *Smilax ornata* (sarsaparilla root). Some women with chronic health problems—for instance, sinusitis—respond to formulas that include anticatarrhals such as *Solidago odorata* (goldenrod herb) or anti-inflammatories such as *Glycyrrhiza glabra* (licorice root).

The herbs that are most useful to enhance natural fertility are the reproductive and nervine relaxants, particularly *Leonurus cardiaca* (motherwort herb), *Scutellaria lateriflora* (skullcap herb), and *Anemone pulsatilla* (pasque flower herb).

Twisted fallopian tubes or an unhealthy uterine lining can be improved with antispasmodics, uterine tissue tonics, and abdominal exercises. A combination of *Caulophyllum thalictroides* (blue cohosh root) and *Cimicifuga racemosa* (black cohosh root) may be the best and simplest herbal way to stimulate tissue health of scarred structures when taken internally. This healing from within may be helped by any one of the many uterine tissue tonics, circulatory tonics, or herbs with an affinity for healthy connective tissue. Choose among them according to their main actions and secondary benefits as described in Chapter 1: Herbal Glossary. It may be helpful to consider *Echinacea spp.* (echinacea root or seed), *Crataegus spp.* (hawthorn leaf, flower, berry) and *Equisetum arvense* (horsetail herb).

Infertility with a hormonal origin responds to herbs that balance the hormone signals, such as *Vitex agnus-castus* (chasteberry seeds), *Angelica sinensis* (dong quai root), and *Trifolium pratense* (red clover blossoms). Other herbs that help would be the nourishing tonics such as *Rubus idaeus* (raspberry leaf) or *Medicago sativa* (alfalfa herb or seed). Herbs with an affinity for the reproductive tract that also have an antimicrobial property to clear infection include *Achillea millefolium* (yarrow). The bitter action of yarrow stimulates the liver to improve general health while metabolizing hormones that are out of balance.

In normal doses, as described in Chapter 2: Herbal Preparation and with each formula below, these herbs pose no health risk during the first few weeks of pregnancy. However, caution is always good practice in pregnancy. As soon as you know you are pregnant, stop taking all herbs that are not specifically recommended or needed during the first three months. Hormones in a woman's body will override most of the common hormonal tonic herbs anyway. It is best to let the body go through its changes without any unnecessary herbal tinkering on our part. Herbs for use during early pregnancy are covered in Chapter 15.

Women can direct their own herbal fertility treatment in the following four stages (please refer to Chapter 1: Herbal Glossary if unfamiliar words appear here):

1. Cleanse the system with alteratives and lymphatics: Formula I.

2. Build up the body's strengths with general tonics, adaptogens, and hormone balancing uterine tonics: Formula II.

3. Stimulate fertility and a healthy reproductive cycle with herbs that have an affinity for reproduction during the follicular phase of the monthly reproductive cycle: Formula III.

4. Stimulate fertility and a healthy reproductive cycle with herbs that have an affinity for reproduction during the luteal phase of the monthly reproductive cycle: Formula IV.

The amount of time a woman needs for cleansing, then rebuilding, depends on her previous health. Each woman is capable of assessing her state of overall health in this regard. Some women who usually take care of their health may need only a week of each stage (cleansing, building, stimulation in the follicular and luteal phases). Other women have more of a backlog of health obstacles.

The average woman usually needs two months for cleansing and rebuilding alone before it makes sense to begin an herbal stimulation phase. If you consider yourself to be out of shape, plan to take cleansing and rebuilding herbs consistently for two months or more before moving on to Formulas III and IV.

As a general guide, divide that time in half: ten to twelve days of cleansing per month (Formula I), followed by ten to twelve days of rebuilding (Formula II). Take a break from herbs during menstrual bleeding. Repeat this for two months or until your cycle is regular and relatively easy. Please don't stop short out of impatience. Patience and a health-conscious routine work wonders.

Cleansing Herbal Formula I for Women

Trifolium pratense (red clover flower)	4 ounces
Calendula officinalis (marigold flower)	3 ounces
Taraxacum officinale (dandelion root)	1 ounce
Taraxacum officinale (dandelion leaf)	1 ounce
Ocimum basilicum (basil leaf)	2 ounces
Equisetum arvense (horsetail herb)	1 ounce

Steep one ounce of herbs in one to two pints of boiling water for twenty minutes; strain. Drink two to four cups a day. In tincture form, take one-half teaspoon in one cup of water three times a day.

Note: Red clover blossoms are often brown, odorless, and useless in commerce; if the ones you find are not fresh-smelling and colorful, see Resources or replace with one ounce of dong quai (*Angelica sinensis*) and three ounces of rose hips (*Rosa spp.*).

Remember, you may use these formulas even if one of the herbs can't be obtained. While the formula is like a "wheel" of herbs designed to roll smoothly, there is still more benefit from taking most of a formula than no herbs at all.

If you are the kind of woman who prefers perfection, you may read about the herb that can't be found, see which actions it brings to the formula, and substitute another appropriate herb listed with that action in Chapter 1: Herbal Glossary. First, find the main action(s) listed there for the herb you cannot get. Then turn to that action category of the Glossary. Select just one herb from that list that seems to fit you and is available. This is fun if you want to learn about herbalism rather than relying on cookbook recipes, as you notice the similarities and differences among plant medicines. Don't overwhelm yourself by looking up every herb; you may not remember even one that way. Start with just the essentials to meet the needs of the present moment.

Building Herbal Formula II for Women

Pfaffia paniculata (suma root)	1 ounce
Vitex agnus-castus (chasteberry seed)	2 ounces
Urtica dioica (nettle leaf)	1 ounce
Rubus idaeus (raspberry leaf)	4 ounces
Leonurus cardiaca (motherwort herb)	½ ounce

Better as tea (standard preparation and dose), this may be combined into one tincture (take 1 teaspoon four times a day). The motherwort tastes bitter and may be replaced with 1 ounce *Anemone pulsatilla* (pasque flower), or you can take motherwort separately as a tincture or extract (½ teaspoon four times a day). For additional information, please see Chapter 2: Herbal Preparation.

Formulas III and IV are stimulating. Formula III is taken during the follicular phase of the reproductive (menstrual) cycle, from the last day of bleeding to ovulation (about ten days to two weeks). Formula IV is taken during the luteal phase, from around ovulation through the first days of bleeding.

Stimulating Herbal Formula III for Women (Follicular Phase)

Angelica sinensis (dong quai)	3 ounces
Panax ginseng (ginseng root)	1 ounce
Eleutherococcus senticosus (Siberian ginseng root)	1 ounce
Smilax ornata (sarsaparilla root)	2 ounces
Turnera diffusa (damiana herb)	3 ounces
Rosmarinus officinalis (rosemary herb)	1 ounce
Cimicifuga racemosa (black cohosh root)	1 ounce

Take as capsules or as extracts combined into one tincture. Tea does not allow the properties of the herbs to work best since many are not fully water-soluble, and the taste is as bad as any formula in this book.

For capsules, grind the herbs, sift the powders together well, and fill #00 capsules. Take three capsules twice a day with meals and a large glass of water.

For tincture, combine the herbs and take one teaspoon three times a day with water (with or without meals).

The first herb in Herbal Formula III is *Angelica sinensis* (dong quai), which stimulates reproductive function before ovulation; once again, more is not better. It has been known to increase bleeding if taken during a menstrual period; this is unnecessary and unhelpful.

The adaptogens in Herbal Formula III for adrenal stress response, nourishing the neurodendocrine pathways, immunity, and blood-sugar stability are ginseng and Siberian ginseng. These make the formula relatively expensive compared to other formulas in this book, but this formula is only taken two weeks a month for one to three months at a time. These stimulating herbs are not taken in large amounts or on their own, but are combined with circulatory tonics and relaxing nervines to encourage mental and emotional equilibrium.

Formula IV balances premenstrual hormones during the second half of the monthly reproductive cycle by replacing dong quai with chasteberry. This herb stimulates healthy function of the corpus luteum. It is combined with antispasmodic *Viburnum opulus* (cramp bark) or the more affordable *Viburnum prunifolium* (black haw bark); one works against reproductive cramping as well as the other in this case.

Formula IV is like a welcome herb garden; it makes a protective circle of tranquillity around this time of the month. It helps a woman through any twinges of PMS, mood changes, and menstrual cramps, and sets the stage for the next ovulation two weeks away. It is not narcotic or sedating, so it does not suppress symptoms, but it can change underlying health.

Stimulating Herbal Formula IV for Women (Luteal Phase)

Vitex agnus-castus (chasteberry)	4 ounces
Viburnum opulus (cramp bark)	1 ounce
Scutellaria lateriflora (skullcap herb)	3 ounces
Panax ginseng (ginseng root)	½ ounce
Eleutherococcus senticosus (Siberian ginseng root)	½ ounce
Smilax ornata (sarsaparilla root)	2 ounces
Rosmarinus officinalis (rosemary herb)	1 ounce

Preparation and dosage are the same as for Formula III.

Depending on your own sense of what you can reasonably do with some consistency, a daily formula may be streamlined to three #00 capsules of Formula IV three times a day. This option saves time but sacrifices the "roundedness" of the four-part health regime described above. The intention of this combination is still to cleanse, rebuild, and tone. It just may happen a little more gradually.

I see couples who are trying herbs and also undergoing the constant stress of fertility tests and artificial insemination. I have no figures or studies to back up this observation, but these people seem slightly less responsive to herbal treatment than those concentrating on natural health, inner serenity, or conventional fertility drug treatment as preparation for conception.

Treatment of the male partner also begins with cleansing and building up the system. With a low sperm count, check for common causes: an undescended testis, drug therapy, chemicals in the workplace, or long hours of sedentary work. Common reasons for low motility (low-energy sperm) include infections (urethritis, chlamydia, gonorrhea) or lack of zinc.

Herbal Formula for Male Partner

Ptychopetalum spp. (muira puama bark)	1 ounce
Panax ginseng (ginseng root)	3 ounces
Eleutherococcus senticosus (Siberian ginseng)	2 ounces
Turnera diffusa (damiana herb)	2 ounces
Mentha spp. (spearmint, peppermint herb)	6 ounces

Prior to preparation, store the first three herbs (the bark and roots) in a separate container from the last two. To prepare, make a standard decoction using ½ ounce of the bark/root mixture in a pint of cold water; cover, bring to a boil, and simmer for thirty minutes. Turn off the heat, add ½ ounce of the mixture of the last two herbs, cover, and steep for fifteen more minutes. Strain and add honey if desired.

To save time, triple the amounts above and store batches in the refrigerator to last three days at a time. Drink one cup twice a day, morning and early evening (it is not as helpful to drink a stimulating brew late in the evening). Drink six days a week, taking a break on the seventh day. Continue for at least 10–12 weeks.

It takes one hour twice a week to make the Herbal Formula for Males. The male partner can make this himself. If he doesn't know how, show him once how to put his herbs in cold water and bring them to a boil. Then let him do his share to nourish the fertile energy between you by keeping up with his tea six days a week. You have enough to do without getting after him to take his herbs.

Muira puama is a safe Brazilian aphrodisiac that may be omitted if it is unavailable in your area (or please see mail-order Suppliers in Appendix). While the African herb *Pausinystalia yohimbe* (yohimbe) has received much press, its popularity is not in proportion to its long-term value for healthy fertility. Its alkaloids are stimulating. Use it at your own discretion and pleasure.

If nervous exhaustion aggravates a male partner's fertility, add:

Rumex crispus (yellow dock root)	½ ounce (to the root portion of the mixture for decoction)
Avena sativa (oat straw herb)	2 ounces

If anemia or low-grade stress are present, add:

Urtica dioica, Urtica spp. (nettle leaf)	2 ounces

If illness or a poor diet precede infertility, add:

Arctium lappa (burdock root)	2 ounces
Verbena officinalis (vervain herb)	⅓ ounce

If there is long-term or severe stress, or if low testosterone levels are found, it may be appropriate to increase ginseng unless an individual also has tension headaches. Add:

Panax ginseng (ginseng root)	2 ounces (for a total of 5 ounces)
Smilax ornata (sarsaparilla root)	2 ounces

Contrary to popular media reports, *neither* of these herbs is an anabolic steroid precursor. Neither is a stimulant to testosterone levels in men or women. Sarsaparilla aids nonspecific immunity (lymphatic function) and endocrine balance in the context of this herbal combination to benefit the *man* (not his testosterone).

Caution: Headaches are one sign of taking excess or unnecessary *Panax ginseng*, though there are many unrelated causes for this common symptom. See an acupuncturist, naturopathic doctor, herbalist, or other care provider regarding extreme fatigue, insomnia, or recurrent headaches.

If infertility is complicated by prostate problems (benign hyperplasia, family history of prostate problems), *Serenoa serrulata* (saw palmetto berry) is an herbal remedy proven safe and effective for men as a reproductive-system tonic. The herb is rich in fatty acids and saponins, so it does not extract well in water. It was used as a fertility-enhancing food by Native Americans of the southeastern United States after droughts or natural disasters reduced their numbers. Saw palmetto is sometimes taken by women as well to improve fertility though it is not recommended in early pregnancy, so I have left it out of women's fertility formulas to be safe.

The oily, soapy taste of saw palmetto berry is not pleasant. One alternative to tea is four #00 capsules twice a day, taken with a glass of milk or after a meal.

Another is to take two teaspoons of tincture with milk or a meal twice a day. This may be taken in addition to the Herbal Formula for Male Partners, six days a week.

Nutrition

Eat a variety of whole foods that remind us of life's cyclical nature and germination. These include eggs, peas, seeds, nuts, fruit with seeds in season, watermelon, pomegranates, figs, zucchini, cooked squash, and other cooked vegetables, from soup to stir-fry.

Plant proteins can be well combined for bioavailable protein, but there is no getting around the fact that meat is stimulating to the human endocrine (hormonal) system. Vegetarians and vegans may have to replace this animal energy through concentrated foods (seeds, nuts, cooked foods).

Nonspecific alterative herbs such as *Urtica dioica* (nettle leaf) and *Arctium lappa* (burdock root) are affordable, even cheap, nourishment added to soups or taken as tea.

Yang food and herbs are helpful to fertility. The macrobiotic use of yin and yang is not identical to the Chinese term which refers to the dynamic half (loosely called "masculine") of an ancient symbol for the cosmic pair of opposites, yin and yang. The word "yang" refers to the sunny side of the mountain: warm, light, charged with a particular quality of dynamic, fiery energy. Things move around a lot on the yang side of the mountain. Yang foods and herbs often grow in these warm conditions (but not always) and carry these qualities. Think of hot chili peppers growing in Southwestern deserts. Nutritionally, women wishing to improve their fertility need a balance of yin and yang foods. Yin foods are soft, cold, and sweet; examples are bread, dairy products, bananas, and even ice cream.

Other Points

Counseling, support groups, and long, hot jasmine–lavender baths before intercourse can make a tremendous difference.

Visualization, or imagining healthy change and conception, has great power. This is not a way of avoiding reality; visualization changes reality. The growing field of energy work may also prove useful in raising internal functions to their ideal level of activity (reiki, polarity, light therapy, or others). From the spiritual to the mundane, we know that our emotions affect our hormones and our hormones affect our fertility.

An "unproven" but helpful suggestion: Walk or exercise out in sunlight without sunglasses/glasses/contacts for a total of about twenty minutes a day. Natural light seems to stimulate the pineal gland in the brain. It is not enough to be out in sunny weather with a car windshield between you and the sun. The pineal gland regulates our biological clock, telling a woman's reproductive system what amount of natural light there is for her to be in alignment with seasonal rhythm, to allow her to start a nine-month pregnancy.

Couples find inspiration from creating rituals of serenity, receptivity, creativity, and intimacy. Together, visualize in great detail the way you want to "see" conception, pregnancy, delivery, and child care. Make room for resolving any parenting or financial concerns that arise. Invest your heart and soul in positive imagery, but be open to reality once you have focused your loving attention on creating your vision. Be relaxed so that you can pay attention to what *is*. Let any judgments fall away.

You might also ask yourselves questions about your vision, purpose, dreams, and desire. What is the purpose of becoming pregnant? To give love? To keep love? Infertility is not necessarily a spiritual or karmic judgment about a couple's "right" to be parents. Infertility is an opportunity for them to understand their own judgments on these matters. There are many ways to mother others. There are many ways to surrender your heart, to create a close-knit healthy family.

15

Pregnancy

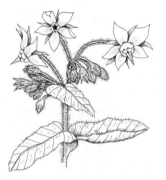

Pregnancy is a powerful and potentially healing time. In this chapter you will first find an explanation of healthy body changes that occur during pregnancy. Second, there is a brief summary of the main herbs that are appropriate to use during pregnancy. Third, "Herbal Tonics for Use During Pregnancy" is a list of tonics for each body system; you may use one or two of these herbs over the long term to prevent constitutional weaknesses from becoming problems. Fourth, "Safe Herbs for Pregnancy and Lactation—A Glossary of Actions" lists herbs with specific properties (gas-relieving, antimicrobial) that are safe to use during pregnancy. Fifth, "Problems of Pregnancy and the Herbs That Treat Them" provides suggestions for treating common problems, from morning sickness to post-partum depression.

Suggestions for natural treatments are followed by "Herbs with Limited Use in Pregnancy," to explain herbs used for special cases only. Finally, there is a list of "Herbs to Avoid During Pregnancy."

When in doubt about your or your baby's health, get a diagnosis from an experienced health care provider before acting on your decision to use a natural treatment.

Definition

Most women who become pregnant understand the basic terms of anatomy and physiology for the reproductive system. There is an egg in the fallopian tube, which orgasmic spasms help move down to meet the sperm; these are moving up the vaginal canal to the fallopian tube in slippery, fertile mucus. With the help of prostaglandins stimulating the fallopian tube's rhythmic muscle waves, a fertilized ovum moves down to settle into the endometrium (the thickened cushion of uterine lining).

Implantation of the fertilized egg occurs four to five days after the sperm meets the egg. One could say this is technically when pregnancy "starts." Even in health, fertilized ova cannot survive to become human beings until implantation connects them to life support: Mother. A baby is one with the mother, feeling her stress or her joy, receiving nourishment from what she puts in her mouth or feels in her heart.

The signals from the fertilized egg keep the corpus luteum in the ovary producing the hormone progesterone: pro-gestation hormone. Progesterone is calming, so it is part of the reason pregnant women feel different emotionally as well as physically. Because progesterone slows down some physiological processes, it can be a cofactor causing symptoms such as constipation, usually relieved by drinking more water rather than taking bowel stimulants.

In the uterus, the developing embryo burrows into the wall, tapping into the mother's blood supply. After the release of HCG, three hormones are produced by cells (*syncytiotrophoblasts*) on the outside of the growing embryo: estrogen, progesterone, and PLG (placental lactogen). PLG is like growth hormone for stimulating fetal development; like prolactin, it causes breast changes in the pregnant woman. More of these syncytiotrophoblasts secure the fetal blood supply from the mother's blood vessels, with a thin membrane between for quick diffusion of food in, waste out. The placenta produces the hormones, which determine the long-term self-regulation of the pregnancy.

Symptoms and Signs

A common symptom of pregnancy is extreme sensitivity to odor, emotional situations, and foods. Morning sickness may come at any time of day, and is usually (but not always) limited to the first trimester.

The obvious way to know that you are pregnant is that your menstrual bleeding is late or never comes, but it is possible to have a little spotting or light flow while pregnant. One out of five pregnant women experience this; if there is continued bleeding or abdominal pain, see your health care provider.

There are women who do not know they are pregnant until close to delivery. These may be intelligent women with little awareness of their bodies, or they may show so little after a history of irregular cycles that it does not occur to them that they have conceived.

Pregnancy is not a disease that herbs have to "fix." The symptoms of common imbalances are signs to take care of oneself. Many symptoms have herbal approaches that tone and relax, encourage and nourish, allowing Nature her way. Every woman is a little different. For millions of pregnant women, herbs have been used in these same ways for a long, long time. However, no words printed on paper, no matter how true, can replace professional health services in person.

For the first two months or so, the baby's growth takes place via hormonal stimulation, then the fetus itself grows and stretches the womb. A woman usually reaches her maximum weight gain by the twentieth week, when the uterine walls begin to thin. Weight gain of twenty to thirty-five pounds is absolutely normal, and encourages us to move slowly and to exercise through and following pregnancy. Obsession with getting back to a pre-pregnancy weight must be balanced with the body's wisdom in holding onto some padding; fat helps cushion hormonal changes after delivery and provides physical cushioning.

The abdominal walls and outer thighs stretch with collagen and elastin changes, making red stripes called *striae gravidarum*, which turn into white stretch marks later.

A nonsteroidal hormone from the placenta, *relaxin*, works with progesterone to soften up the joints of bones, especially between the two halves of the pelvic bone structures, to allow the baby to pass through the birth canal. This is why pregnant women have lower back pain, sciatica, and problems with their hips and knees.

Breasts enlarge and become sensitive by the second month to the point where pressure from clothes hurts. Increased blood supply shows as blue veins, while the areola around the nipple deepens in color; the secondary ring around the areola also develops and remains after pregnancy. *Colostrum* (the milk produced just before and after delivery) is made in breasts as early as the tenth week, thanks to progesterone and estrogen levels. The breast milk ducts develop into branched tubes until they are ready by the twentieth week.

The lungs adjust to pregnancy by increasing the rate of respiration as the diaphragm experiences pressure, giving shallower breaths and sometimes a slightly breathless quality. This is one way the body insists on moving more slowly rather than allowing a woman to keep running around, working late, as if she is not pregnant. Though immunity and many aspects of health are optimal during a woman's pregnancies due to extra care on her part, there is an increased tendency to get respiratory infections.

The kidney and bladder experience the pressure of a growing baby throughout pregnancy under the influence of an orchestra of hormones. Complex changes including increased blood flow to the kidneys and bladder may show up hidden problems with kidneys or simple increase of bladder function. Frequency of urination has caused many a pregnant woman to rearrange her life around her proximity to the nearest rest room. When the bladder cannot always empty completely due to pressure, bladder infections become an added nuisance.

Digestion is affected by pregnancy, and not just in terms of morning sickness. Heartburn is simply a sign of a woman's increased sensitivity to foods, changes in stomach acidity, and the stomach contents being squished by the growing fetus.

In the digestive system of a pregnant woman, there is also an increase in saliva and acidity of the saliva, which is behind the old folk belief that for every child a woman loses a tooth due to increased calcium demand and acid pH. It is not unusual for women to experience dental problems or sore gums during these nine months. Excessive saliva (*ptyalism*) may occur during the second trimester, though anxiety may be associated with the hormonal changes behind this.

This is not the time to indulge in ice cream and French fries, though odd cravings are said to characterize our pregnancies. Many cravings are sound, but when a woman craves irritating low-quality foods, it may be a sign of her need to stimulate or kick-start homeostasis.

Cause

Whether through heterosexual intercourse or technologically assisted fertilization, implantation of the fertilized ovum is the starting point of pregnancy.

Conventional Medical Care

Gynecologists and obstetricians tend to focus on potential complications of pregnancy rather than on health. This is understandable from people who train and work in a place where very sick people go. Unless there are problems, there is very little treatment other than pre-natal care: education, nutritional advice, and monitoring.

Herbal Treatment

In this section, I will provide basic information about the herbs frequently recommended to treat common problems of pregnancy. Not all the medicinal plants that can be used during pregnancy appear here. Some that I have left out are endangered, such as *Chamaelirium luteum* (false unicorn root). Some are not part of my personal experience but are used effectively by other herbalists; *Gossypium spp.* (cotton root bark) for example. These "pregnancy herbs" are frequently used to encourage a good term and labor.

When it comes to herbs for pregnancy, it is usually better to use teas, not alcohol tinctures. Though alcohol content may be diminished by adding boiling water to a cup containing a dose of herbal tincture, it does not evaporate all the alcohol. It is safe to use some tinctures nearer the end of term because of convenience and quicker action. But women who desire to be absolutely safe should rely on herb teas. Our bodies are designed in pregnancy to respond well to herbs and water. Glycerin tinctures are just slightly laxative and may also affect blood sugar. In pregnancy, this isn't always a bad thing, but a limit of two teaspoons of glycerin tincture is a safe, conservative dose.

The list of teas is arranged from the most popular or commonly-relied-upon herbs to those with specific uses. These herbs may be used singly or in combination.

Rubus idaeus (raspberry leaf) is taken as tea, made in the usual way: one glass two to three times a day. It is safe to take and is recommended during the first two trimesters. This is done, at the least, throughout the last trimester. It is often made up in a large batch to keep on hand throughout labor for sipping. Since it isn't often convenient to drink a lot (and then have to get up more often) during delivery, this tea can be poured into ice cube trays, then broken up into small ice chips to suck on when the mouth feels dry. This feels more comfortable for women, and prevents drinking tea which leads to a full bladder, requiring trips to the bathroom. Raspberry leaf coordinates uterine contractions for an easier birth, making it the best "partus preparation" (prepares one for labor and/or delivery).

Mitchella repens (partridgeberry or squaw vine herb) is an herb used by Native American midwives. It is used throughout the third trimester the same as raspberry or in combination with raspberry when there have been difficulties with pregnancies in the past. The dose is limited to one cup of tea of the single herb per day or up to one-fourth part of a formula by weight, three standard cups per day. Partridgeberry herb does apparently contradictory things: It relaxes pregnant women while it tones up the uterine and pelvic muscles, and it soothes nervous "jumpiness." Its actions are: astringent (for weak uterine tone, but it is not drying or constipating), diuretic, emmenagogue (especially in ill health or in larger doses than described here), and *parturient* (helps with labor and delivery) taken during the few weeks before birth.

Caulophyllum thalictroides (blue cohosh root) is only taken if needed. As a uterine tonic, it is used in earlier stages of pregnancy to prevent miscarriages, when it acts as an antispasmodic. It may also be used in delivery after labor has begun if there is stalled labor accompanied by fatigue. The dose in early pregnancy is one and a half cups of the decoction daily. During labor, it is more convenient to use tincture, up to one-half teaspoon per dose; directions are given more fully in "Herbs with

Limited Use in Pregnancy." A woman usually knows if her pregnancy is unstable or her health is out of balance. Blue cohosh may "normalize health" by bringing on a period (the action: emmenagogue). It contains steroidal saponins, which are anti-inflammatory.

Cimicifuga racemosa (black cohosh root) is a tonic to the uterus as well as a relaxing nervine, so it paradoxically relaxes muscular tension, including painfully cramping pregnant uterine muscle. This is useful when there are problems with threatened miscarriage in the first or second trimester. Otherwise this herb is only used at the end of pregnancy, as a tincture in half-teaspoon doses.

When a threatened miscarriage (or a history of them) indicates use of black cohosh earlier in pregnancy, the dose is one and a half cups of decoction per day or one-fourth part by weight of a combination, three standard cups per day. If tissue is tight, it may not be in good tone, so these actions are not as contradictory in pregnancy as it may appear. Black cohosh contains phytoestrogens that promote estrogen, but hormonal feedback mechanisms of the pregnant human female are stronger.

Capsella bursa-pastoris (shepherd's purse) is a safe astringent for spotting or bleeding at any stage during pregnancy, though it cannot stop a miscarriage. It has saponins and mustard oils while the peptide fraction makes it oxytoxic (stimulating to unterine contractions). It is one of the preparations that is always made from fresh herb, never dried. It is particularly meant for treating blood in the urine (the cause must be diagnosed), including kidney or bladder infections that are severe enough to cause blood loss from chronic inflammation. There is no toxic dose of the fresh tincture indicated in the literature, and the safe dose is the effective dose as long as the causes for bleeding are being attended to even if the herb stops the symptom of blood loss.

Anemone pulsatilla (pasque flower herb) is better made (tea, tincture, or powdered capsules) from dried herb in pregnancy due to *emodin* content. Pasque flower is an antispasmodic, a pain-reliever, and a nervine relaxant, though it is stimulating to blood circulation. It is taken in standard doses, but for severe pain that has been diagnosed and attended to, doses of up to five (four-ounce) glasses of tea per day or six half-teaspoons of tincture may be augmented with other treatment for pain relief, including foot massage and bed rest.

Zea mays (corn silk thread) consists of the thin, pale yellow strands between corn on the cob and the outer green husks saved from summer crops of organic corn. They dry in a day for storage. Tea from home-dried organic corn silk is more effective than commercial brown corn silk. If it has no aroma or sweet flavor, tea or tincture of the herb will not work well. This herb tea is the safest soothing demulcent for cystitis (inflamed bladder or bladder infection), common in pregnancy.

The extra fluid of tea also makes this form of preparation more appropriate in pregnancy.

The plant starches in corn silk are osmotic diuretics. That means that the starches stay in the urine instead of being absorbed in the body, and they act like magnets for water. This draws water from swollen ankles or puffy areas under the skin into the kidneys and bladder, washing out bacteria in the increased stream of urine. The corn silk starches are not like refined, simple sugars that worsen kidney and bladder infections by supplying bacteria with instant fuel. They feel soothing to an inflamed bladder and urethra. No toxicity is known, so the limiting factor is how much tea a woman can drink until she feels relief, usually two to six cups over a day or two. Corn silk works well as a simple infusion, but also combines well with marshmallow root, another safe osmotic diuretic during pregnancy.

Trillium erectum (bethroot or birthroot) is listed in all the books as a pregnancy herb, but it is now endangered. If you live where it is locally plentiful (the Midwest and parts of the East Coast), you may use it with less concern. It is a great uterine tonic, especially near the end of term when contraction begins. It promotes a short, speedy labor.

No one formula works for everyone, so mix and match for yourself if you prefer, using herbs noted for their safety and their effects that would benefit you. The combinations that follow are intended to be helpful and harmless in the hands of a novice, but a careful reader or a trained herbalist can pick and choose from other information in this book.

Pregnancy is not the best time for experiments. When a pregnant women is in doubt about trying a perfect-sounding herb she has no experience with, it is best to ask an herbalist or a natural health care provider about it first.

Everyone responds to herbs a little differently. This is especially relevant during the first trimester when women and herbs interact in sometimes unpredictable ways due to their extreme sensitivity. In pregnancy the senses are heightened so that a woman can know right away whether or not a substance or experience is helpful to mother and child. Listen to the wisdom of your body.

Fresh herb tea is the best form for all of these herbs to avoid any irritation from hard-to-digest capsules and powders or alcohol tinctures.

The blood supply that nourishes the baby is from the mother's own blood supply. Alteratives, or "blood cleansers," and gentle tonics help build up the mother's nutrition, dietary assimilation, and healthy elimination. Two appropriate examples are burdock root and nettle leaf. Safe and effective hepatics (herbs that help the liver) are dandelion leaf and root and milk thistle seed. The latter is especially helpful if there have been liver problems in the past, such as hepatitis, drug use, or alcohol.

Herbal Formula I

Rubus idaeus (raspberry leaf)	3 ounces
Tilia spp. (linden flower, leaf)	1 ounce
Taraxacum officinalis (dandelion root)	2 ounces
Taraxacum officinalis (dandelion leaf)	1 ounce

Standard infusion: one tablespoon of herb mixture in one and a half pints of water. Any herb for flavor may be added; choose one or two that agree with you from those listed in "Safe Herbs for Pregnancy and Lactation." Add more water until flavor is mild enough for a sensitive palate.

In Herbal Formula I, which is for general prevention and health, raspberry is a toning astringent as well as a "uterine preparator" (prepares the uterus for labor); linden is a mild relaxant nervine and a cardiovascular system tonic; dandelion is a hepatic and mineral-rich diuretic. Together they have a cleansing effect. An additional alterative is not needed unless a woman is in need of deep tissue cleansing from dietary or other toxins.

To help manage or prevent problems with high blood pressure, pregnant women will benefit from a formula that incorporates a cardiovascular tonic herb such as hawthorn, which also lowers high blood pressure. To relax the smooth muscle surrounding constricted blood vessels (and other tight muscles in the body), a vasodilator and antispasmodic such as cramp bark is helpful. Because stress and indigestion often play a role in high blood pressure, a nervine that is soothing to digestion is linden. Another nervine tonic that calms the mind and emotions is skullcap; this combines well with dandelion, a nutritive, mineralizing diuretic that decreases water retention without depleting a woman's store of electrolytes.

Herbal Formula II

Rubus idaeus (raspberry leaf)	3 ounces
Crataegus spp. (hawthorn flower, leaf, and berry)	3 ounces
Viburnum opulus (cramp bark)	1 ounce
Tilia spp. (linden flower)	1 ounce
Scutellaria spp. (skullcap herb)	1 ounce
Taraxacum officinalis (dandelion leaf)	1 ounce

Use a minimum of one teaspoon of herb mixture to one cup of water, and a maximum of one ounce of herbs to a pint and a half of water, steeped for fifteen minutes (see Chapter 2: Herbal Preparation if more information is needed); strain and drink one cup three times a day, or sip throughout the day.

Add any herb for taste from "Safe Herbs for Pregnancy and Lactation," but do not use sugar or artificial sweetener. Licorice root might seem like a good choice for flavor, and it may be fine for some pregnant women, but with others it may cause a rise in blood pressure due to its effects on water retention. Avoid licorice root in cases of gestational hypertension.

Herbal Tonics for Use During Pregnancy

There are many possible herbs to use during pregnancy, but these are among the safest preventive herbs for common problems in each body system. You can use one or two of these tonics for their specific properties as you like, added to an herbal formula or taken separately as needed.

Digestive System   meadowsweet herb, dandelion leaf and root, lemon balm herb, chamomile flower, lemon juice in water

Cardiovascular System   hawthorn berries, linden blossom

Respiratory System   mullein leaf and flower, elder flower, sweet violet leaf and flower

Urinary Tract   eight glasses of water daily, ten ounces of unsweetened cranberry juice diluted in water daily, corn silk "hair" tea (from organic corn; dry between two paper towels for a day and store in a tin, glass jar, or brown paper bag for up to four months)

Nervous System   oatmeal and oat straw herb, skullcap herb, passionflower herb, chamomile herb, catnip herb, lavender flower, motherwort herb, and damiana leaf (not root). Of the last two listed, take only one-half cup of tea daily in small doses.

Muscles and Bones   horsetail herb, meadowsweet herb, burdock root, raspberry leaf

Endocrine or Hormonal System   bladderwrack seaweed, kelp seaweed, nettle leaf, blueberry leaf and fruit

Skin   elder flower, dandelion root and leaf, nettle leaf (of nettles, take only one-half cup of tea daily)

Immune System   shiitake mushrooms, reishi mushrooms, echinacea root and seeds, garlic cloves (garlic is very safe, but it may give newly pregnant women digestive gas). Reishi mushrooms must be decocted (standard preparation) to get their immune properties. The does is ½ cup a day, alone or with other herbs.

Safe Herbs for Pregnancy and Lactation—A Glossary of Actions

Herbs marked with an asterisk (*) are for limited use or external use, as described.

Adaptogens help relieve long-term stress:
borage flower, nettle leaf

Alteratives are used for detoxification:
nettle leaf, red clover flower, alfalfa herb, lemon grass leaf, rose hips fruit, cleavers herb

Analgesics relieve the symptom of pain:
valerian root, passionflower herb, lavender flower, cabbage leaves* (externally for mastitis)

Antidepressants help lift the heart and spirit:
vervain herb, lemon balm herb, lavender flower, borage flower, lemon verbena leaf and flower

Antiemetics lessen vomiting and morning sickness:
black horehound herb, raspberry leaf, lemon balm herb, chamomile flower, ginger root. (Of ginger, take sips as needed, up to one-half cup of tea daily.)

Anti-inflammatories reduce inflammation without suppressing symptoms:
chamomile flower, meadowsweet herb, St. Johnswort herb, wild yam root (one-half cup of tea daily)

Antimicrobials help natural defenses clear infections:
garlic clove (internally for general immunity, infections of the lungs, or digestion), shiitake mushrooms, corn silk (for painful urinary-tract infections), echinacea root (always safe internally for viral or bacterial infections and low immunity), thyme herb* (limit to two half-cups of tea a day for three days; used internally for lungs and digestion, externally for skin), uva-ursi leaf*, goldenseal root* (externally on wounds only), myrrh resin* (externally on infections or burns only), ti tree essential oil* (externally on yeast, fungal, or other surface infections only)

Antispasmodics slow or stop smooth and skeletal muscle spasms such as cramps:
cramp bark, black haw bark (uterine spasms), valerian root (nervous muscle cramping), chamomile flower (intestinal spasms)

Aperients and **laxatives** relieve congestion in the pelvic region due to sluggish bowel. Note: Stronger herbs sold as laxatives may stimulate uterine contractions; try plain water or these gentle tonics first:

dandelion root, one-fourth cup of prunes (soaked dried fruit), flax seed, psyllium seed. After trying these, you may use the stronger yellow dock root (one-half cup daily for one to three days if needed).

Astringents stem excess flow of fluids such as heavy bleeding or discharge:

yarrow, witch hazel bark, periwinkle, pasque flower herb, partridgeberry herb (one-half cup of tea daily)

Bitters work on dyspepsia, gas, constipation, hemorrhoids, hypoglycemia, depression, digestive health, and physical energy. Note: Stronger bitters than these may be oxytocic, stimulating uterine contractions along with intestinal movement, so avoid mugwort and other bitters or laxatives not listed in this section:

chicory root, dandelion root and leaf, chamomile flower, burdock root

Carminatives dispel gas:

peppermint leaf, fennel seed, anise seed, dill seed, ginger root, chamomile flower, caraway seed

Demulcents soothe raw, irritated membranes or skin, internally or externally:

marshmallow root, slippery elm bark powder, corn silk, aloe* (external use for burns, scrapes)

Diuretics increase urine output, reducing water retention:

dandelion leaf, marshmallow, corn silk

Galactogogues increase the flow of breast milk:

fennel seed, anise seed, milk thistle seed, and vervain herb after delivery

Hepatics resolve constipation, metabolize hormones, aid elimination, help skin problems, and improve digestion of fats:

dandelion root, lemon juice in water

Hormonal normalizers affect feedback loops to balance the sex hormones naturally (after delivery for strength and recuperation, post-partum depression, or before conception to promote regular cycle):

red clover flower, chasteberry, and dong quai

Labor tonics strengthen and prepare the reproductive organs for delivery:

raspberry leaf, partridgeberry*, black* and blue cohoshes* (see "Herbs with Limited Use in Pregnancy")

Oxytocics stimulate uterine contractions. First try increasing intake of water, waiting for the baby to be ready, nourishment of body and soul, and even exercise alternating with bed rest. Then consider using one of these with an experienced midwife's or herbalist's assistance. For directions on use, please see "Herbs with Limited Use in Pregnancy". Note: None of these are recommended for herbal abortions. Herbs are not safe means of stimulating a successful termination: blue cohosh root*, black cohosh root* (often in equal parts; see "Long or Stalled Labor")

Nervine relaxants synergize with antispasmodics and analgesics to reduce anxiety, irritability, and tension:
chamomile flower, skullcap herb, valerian root, passionflower herb, lemon balm herb

Nervine tonics help restore healthy tissue and functioning of nerves after stress to leave you in better shape:
oat straw and food, St. Johnswort flower, skullcap herb

Vulneraries may be taken internally but are usually placed externally to heal tears, wounds, burns, and abrasions—wherever we are *vulnerable*—by knitting epithelial cells together with little or no scarring:
comfrey root and leaf* (externally and vaginally only during pregnancy), chamomile flower, plantain leaf, St. Johnswort flower

Problems of Pregnancy and the Herbs That Treat Them

Many common problems of pregnancy may respond to natural remedies, from the time when a woman notices she hasn't had a period to the time when the baby is starting to crawl.

There are so many herbs available that it can be overwhelming trying to decide what to use when one needs something "right now." Below are several conditions that respond to specific herbs, combinations of herbs, or simple home remedies.

Some of the following conditions are self-limiting—they may clear up without any treatment. Some require a licensed health care provider to diagnose and possibly treat the problem. Yet natural approaches may help women return to full health with fewer medications, side effects, and expense. When integrated medicine using natural remedies at home may not be sufficient, cautions are given.

Any flowering herb or natural substance may cause problems for some people, but all of these are considered traditional standbys for safety and effectiveness. If there is a worsening of any condition when using any herb, the mother or baby may have an individual reaction and the herb should be discontinued and noted as something for that individual to avoid. These are listed in the order that they typically occur during pregnancy.

Morning Sickness   Have: complex carbohydrate at bedside, more water, protein, pre-natal multivitamins, vitamin-B complex

Avoid: fried foods, antihistamines, nausea medications

Try: antinausea herbs such as ginger or black horehound herb (Note: This is *Ballota nigra*, *not* the more common white horehound, *Marrubium vulgare*). Use as a standard tea (see Chapter 2: Herbal Preparation), flavored with honey or these more delicious antinausea herbs (use alone or in any combination to taste): peppermint, lemon balm, chamomile, raspberry, ginger (cup of tea daily), peach leaf

Heartburn   Have: small frequent meals, regular exercise (at least a slow walk after meals)

Avoid: rich fatty foods, curries, cakes, black tea/coffee, cold orange or grapefruit juice

Try: demulcent teas to reduce excess stomach acid (any one or more of peppermint, spearmint, lemon balm, meadowsweet, marshmallow)

Diarrhea   Have: applesauce with dash of powdered cinnamon, soups, barley with a dash of powdered cayenne

Avoid: stress, badly prepared foods, dairy products

Try: apples (the pectin is binding for diarrhea, while the fiber acts as a bulk laxative for constipation), a standard preparation of meadowsweet or chamomile tea

Constipation   Have: little or no red meat and dairy products, two apples a day, one-half cup cooked whole grains four times a week, steamed or raw vegetables, four ounces of prune juice diluted with equal parts water daily as needed, one teaspoon of fresh lemon juice in eight ounces of water before bedtime (empty bladder last thing at night), one to two teaspoons of bulk fiber (flax, psyllium seeds) followed by two large glasses of water

Avoid: excess bread, carbohydrates, dairy products, red meat

Try: a mild bitter (dandelion) and/or a carminative to help relieve or prevent intestinal gas pains (ginger, fennel, dill, chamomile). Use one ounce of herb(s) per pint of water, steep covered for fifteen minutes; strain tea and drink one cup of herb tea a day for five days.

Hemorrhoids   Have: eight glasses of water, herb tea, or juice a day; easily digested food; two days of low-protein in the diet

Avoid: straining at bowel movements, heavy lifting, excess meat, dairy products, spicy food

Try: Kegel exercises (please consult your health care provider for instructions). If hemorrhoids cause a burning sensation, apply cold compresses of distilled witch hazel extract externally.

If hemorrhoids are bleeding, use one of the following, externally: witch hazel, comfrey, plantain, periwinkle, or oak bark. Take one-fourth ounce of dried herb, grind into a powder, stir in with six tablespoons of olive or herb oil (see Chapter 2: Herbal Preparation or "Preventing Tears," later in this section). "Digest" the herb and oil together (on low heat for four hours or overnight); strain while warm through muslin or cheesecloth. Pour into small saucepan with two to three teaspoons (approximately ½–¾ ounce) of shaved or chipped beeswax; add six drops each of chamomile and ti tree essential oils. Let cool to solidify into a salve. Apply before and after bowel movements; wash hands well with each use.

For quick relief, try an echinacea and comfrey sitz bath (one pint of each tea in a hot shallow bath covering buttocks, thighs, and lower back). Soak for fifteen to thirty minutes, adding hot water to tolerance. Repeat once a night for three nights, but expect symptom relief after one soak.

Varicose Veins   Have: beets, buckwheat, whole grains, rest with legs elevated

Avoid: constipation

Try: one to two cups of tea daily for three weeks minimum (standard preparation), using one or more of the following: gingko, dandelion, witch hazel bark (not distilled witch hazel from the drugstore, which is to be used externally only). For flavor, add any herbs from "Safe Herbs for Pregnancy and Lactation."

Water Retention   Have: more water—really! (It acts as a diuretic.) Small amounts of parsley (¼ ounce fresh or 2 teaspoons dried every three days) in salads, in soups, or chopped and added on top of cooked grains.

Avoid: dairy products, salt (including "health food" salt—sea salt, gomasio, tamari), caffeine, strong herbal diuretics (uva ursi, juniper)

Try: one to two cups of tea (standard preparation), using dandelion leaf, corn silk, or both

Cystitis   Have: "live" yogurt; eight to twelve ounces of unsweetened cranberry juice diluted with an equal amount of water; barley water (cook ¼ cup barley in 3 cups water and drink; can add cooked barley to soups); one gram (1,000 milligrams) of vitamin C daily

Avoid: sugar, glucose-sweetened cranberry juice

Try: one to four cups of tea (standard preparation) a day for three days, using one of the following: corn silk, marshmallow, horsetail

If there is much pain or spasm with a bladder infection, use the following herb tea:

Zea mays (corn silk)	2 ounces
Viburnum opulus (cramp bark)	2 ounces
Althaea officinalis (marshmallow root, leaf)	2 ounces
Cinnamomum spp. (cinnamon bark)	¼ ounce

Steep one ounce of herb mixture in a pint of water for fifteen minutes; strain and drink one cup three times a day for three to five days.

As a last resort before taking antibiotics for cystitis, make a tea of *Zea mays* (corn silk), one ounce to four cups standard infusion. To each cup, add one teaspoon of echinacea tincture, and one-fourth teaspoon of *Capsella bursa-pastoris* (shepherd's purse) tincture, even without symptoms of spotting or blood in the urine. CAUTION: Shepherd's purse may be stimulating to the uterus, so do not use it in larger amounts or without genuine need. Many women have used it without a problem, but it is optional; omit it if there are contractions or problems with the pregnancy other than minor spotting due to cystitis. If there is no improvement in that time (3–5 days), don't use more; see your care provider.

Colds, Flus, Sore Throats, Infections   Have: one to five grams of vitamin C daily, a daily gargle with one-half teaspoon of sea salt in water (try not to swallow too much; you don't need extra salt), one to three cloves of garlic in food per day for two to ten days, one-half teaspoon of powdered ginger root or a one-inch piece of ginger root chopped in stir-fried vegetables, shiitake mushrooms in food two nights a week for one to three weeks, lavender essential oil foot baths, extra rest

Avoid: cold draughts, late nights, public places

Try: for flu, two to four cups of hot peppermint and elder tea in equal parts (standard combination) with fresh lemon and honey to taste.

For sore throats, gargle with *Salvia officinalis* var. *purpurea* (red sage) tea or *Commiphora spp.* (myrrh) tincture diluted in honey and water—don't swallow.

For general infections, take one teaspoon of echinacea tincture or one cup of tea (standard preparation) four times a day for two to ten days.

Anemia   (Please see additional information in Chapter 7) Have: liver twice a week if you are not a vegetarian, blackstrap molasses, nuts, culinary amounts of parsley herb (no more than ¼ ounce fresh or 2 teaspoons dried every three days), kelp or other seaweeds one to two times a week, food-source liquid iron supplements (such as Floradix; also see "Maid of Iron" formula in Chapter 7: Iron Deficiency Anemia).

Try: one cup of tea (standard preparation), using one or more of the following: yellow dock, nettles, red clover, alfalfa, rose hips

Low Calcium, Causing Mouth, Teeth, and Gum Problems Have: almonds, nuts, seeds, leafy green vegetables, whole grains, possibly dairy products unless otherwise indicated (malabsorption syndrome, food allergies); have a check-up with a dentist or physician

Avoid: excess salt or protein (leaches calcium from body), hard candy, cold fruit from refrigerator

Try: sea salt gargles, eating garlic, herbal mouthwash (don't swallow too much), using one or more of: echinacea, thyme, chamomile, mint, oak bark (as tea or tinctures diluted in water)

Insomnia Have: a long talk with someone, a great book to read (try children's literature, spiritual writings), more exercise during the day, a relaxing massage, a warm bath or shower with lavender (for a shower, put the lavender on a washcloth or a few drops in the shower stall)

Avoid: caffeine, soft drinks, chocolate, disturbing media imagery

Try: two hot cups of relaxing nervine tea before sleep:

Herbal Formula

Scutellaria spp. (skullcap herb)	3 ounces
Avena sativa (oats, oat straw herb)	1 ounce
Matricaria recutita (chamomile flower)	2 ounces
Tilia spp. (linden flower)	1 ounce
Passiflora incarnata (passionflower herb)	2 ounces
Zingiber officinale (ginger root)	¼ ounce, to taste

Ginger is optional. Steep 1½ ounces of herb mixture in 3½ cups of water, covered, for fifteen minutes; strain tea. Drink one cup two hours before bed, the second cup a half-hour before bed (empty your bladder last thing at night). You may drink more as needed.

Cramps Have: deep breathing to increase oxygen in the blood; moderate physical exercise balanced with rest; calcium in the diet from almonds, nuts, and green leafy and root vegetables

Avoid: heavy lifting, cold places, quick movement

Try: one to two teaspoons of tincture every fifteen minutes as needed, or one cup of tea (standard preparation), repeated as needed, using one or more of the following: cramp bark, black haw, skullcap, valerian

Aches and Pains   Have: weekly prenatal massage, possibly with relaxing essential oils (lavender, chamomile, rose); regular exercise

Avoid: excess red meat, refined sugar

Try: one to three cups of tea daily as needed (standard preparation), using one or more of: skullcap, willow, birch bark, meadowsweet

Gestational Diabetes   Have: a check-up with your health care provider. This is a serious condition requiring medical attention, so inform your care provider if you want to incorporate alternative treatment.

Attend to nutrition first. Incorporate at least a few of the foods believed to stabilize or lower excess blood glucose on a daily basis, such as bitter salad vegetables (endive, escarole, radicchio).

Attend to stress second (for more information, please see "Adaptogens" in Chapter 1: Herbal Glossary).

Try: frequent small tastes of gentian tincture as needed, or one-half teaspoon of devil's club root tincture (*Oplopanax horridum*, not *Harpagophytum procumbens*, devil's claw), diluted in water before meals.

Suma (*Pfaffia paniculata*), a Brazilian root, is an adaptogen used only after the first trimester for balancing blood sugar, or for malnourished South American pregnant women living in city ghettos. It is available as powder in capsules. After the fifth month, use 2 #00 capsules with meals and water twice a day.

Weight Gain   Have: prenatal activity, two pieces of fresh fruit a day, complex whole foods in the diet (normal weight gain is 28–36 pounds)

Avoid: salt, refined sugar, excess red meat, dairy products, foods high in fat, "herbal weight loss" products (they are usually based on diuretics or laxatives that are unsafe during pregnancy)

Try:

Althaea officinalis (marshmallow root)	1 ounce
Matricaria recutita (chamomile flower)	1 ounce
Urtica dioica (nettle leaf)	½ ounce
Elettaria cardamomum (cardamom pods, seeds)	½ ounce

Take one cup of tea (standard preparation) two times a day before or in between meals for two to ten days.

Headache   Have: water, a piece of fruit, a neck-and-shoulder rub, naps, good lighting in work or reading areas, foot baths of lavender essential oil (if headaches are frequent or severe, see your health care provider)

Avoid: cleaning products, fumes, heavy traffic, waiting too long between meals, dehydration, violent movies, the evening news, aspirin, over-the-counter pain relievers

Try: cool compresses of tea made with equal parts rosemary and lavender; massaging two to three drops of essential oil into your temples and the back of your neck, using one or more of: eucalyptus, peppermint, spearmint, lemon balm, rosemary, lavender; a weak half-cup of coffee

Sore Breasts   Have: loose cotton clothing

Avoid: tight bras, caffeine, salt

Try: castor oil or linseed (flax seed) poultices (see Chapter 2: Herbal Preparation).

If breast tenderness accompanies mastitis (inflammation of breast tissue), during pregnancy or breast-feeding, take one teaspoon of echinacea tincture internally and apply cabbage-and-potato poultices externally to help relieve pain and stimulate lymphatic drainage. Take two to three outer cabbage leaves and pound the thick middle rib until pliable, or chop coarsely. Grate one-quarter of a potato and add it to the cabbage. Add just enough hot water to mix well and let the mixture cool to a comfortable temperature; apply wet leaves or vegetable mash to breasts. Cover with a dry towel for twenty to sixty minutes. Repeat one to two times a day for two to three days, as needed.

Sore Nipples   Have: air baths, rough towels (to toughen up tender skin), self-massage, a breast pump if unable to feed baby temporarily

Avoid: breast-feeding on the worst side for a day

Try: external salves of comfrey, calendula, plantain, and/or St. Johnswort. Many salves are available commercially that will work just fine, or see Chapter 2: Herbal Preparation. Apply several times a day; wipe clean with a dry cloth before feeding, then reapply several times daily for three to seven days as needed.

Preventing Tears and Episiotomies   Have: exercise in prenatal program

Try: massaging an herbal oil into your external genitalia and perineal area nightly. Use four ounces of olive or sesame oil to "digest" (at the lowest possible heat, overnight or for up to a week) 1½ ounces of one or more of following: comfrey leaf, St. Johnswort, calendula. Strain through muslin or cheesecloth. Add 10 drops of tincture of benzoin (available from drugstores) or lavender essential oil as a preservative; store in a clean jar with a tight-fitting lid. Massage 1 teaspoon into the perineum once or twice day for at least the last trimester, preferably the whole term. By the ninth month, the perineum feels well lubricated and elastic, and has a good blood supply. Mothers report results ranging from no tears to small tears that heal quickly. More than stitches, this and Kegel exercises ensure a quick return of pleasure in sexuality after giving birth.

Bleeding   Have: a diagnosis from your health care provider unless it is an obvious external wound or a minor bleed. One-fifth of pregnant women experience a little spotting. Only half of these lose the pregnancy. If in doubt, or if fever, pain, or nausea develops, get checked first. In the first or second trimester, try *Rubus idaeus* (raspberry leaf) tea in standard preparations plus ½ teaspoon *Capsella bursa-pastoris* (shepherd's purse) tincture every four hours.

Avoid: excess activity

Try: in the third trimester, the following tea for internal use:

Anemone pulsatilla (pasque flower herb)	3 ounces
Mitchella repens (partridgeberry herb)	½ ounce
Quercus spp. (oak bark)	1 ounce
Cinnamomum spp. (cinnamon bark)	½ ounce

Cinnamon is optional. Decoct 1 ounce of herb mixture on low heat for 20 minutes; strain tea and drink ½ cup of tea every hour until bleeding subsides.

To heal perineum tears (see "Preventing Tears and Episiotomies," page 161), apply comfrey tea compresses (strained tea, comfortable temperature, on clean dry cotton or soft flannel). If pressure applied longer than five to fifteen minutes is required to staunch bleeding, hold the compress firmly while someone calls your health care provider or other professional medical help.

Herpes   Have: overall good nutrition, regular exercise for reducing stress level (a trigger for outbreaks), and a positive attitude. Send yourself on a holiday perhaps with your partner, even if it's just a few hours at home with the other kids away and the door closed.

Eat foods rich in beta-carotene and lysine; take vitamins A, B, and C .

If practical, eat one to three cloves of raw garlic daily (up to individual taste; this is optional).

Try: the following combination, which is safe during pregnancy:

Rubus idaeus (raspberry leaf)	3 ounces
Avena sativa (oat straw herb)	2 ounces
Echinacea spp. (echinacea root)	4 ounces
Anemone pulsatilla (pasque flower; flower, herb)	2 ounces
Melissa officinalis (lemon balm herb)	4 ounces
Scutellaria lateriflora (skullcap herb)	1 ounce

Steep 1 ounce of this mixture in 2 pints of boiling water for 20 minutes; strain tea. Drink one 12–16-ounce glass a day, for a minimum of two weeks. For longer-term use if needed, drop the echinacea to 2 ounces. Continue for one to three months as needed; consultation with your health care provider and an herbalist is advisable. Note: Since pregnant women are sensitive to flavor, lemon balm is optional; it is considered antiviral, it settles digestive upsets, and it tastes good to most pregnant women.

Treat your partner with the formula just described; if your partner is male, add 1 ounce each of: saw palmetto, damiana, and baptisia.

Threatened Abortion   Have: immediate medical attention, bed rest. Vaginal bleeding in the first half of term, with serious uterine cramping and backache, requires a licensed health care provider. In addition, herbs may be important to the health of the mother and baby.

Try:

Dioscorea villosa (wild yam root)	1 ounce
Mitchella repens (partridgeberry herb)	1 ounce
Viburnum opulus (cramp bark)	3 ounces
Viburnum prunifolium (black haw bark)	3 ounces

Decoct 3 ounces of herb mixture in 1 quart of water for 20 minutes; strain and drink 1 wine glassful (⅓–½ cup or 3–4 ounces) every two to four hours until symptoms cease.

Abortion is inevitable if membranes break and the cervix dilates. Your health care provider can check. These symptoms, whether or not there is fever or passed material, require medical attention to prevent infection, pelvic inflammatory disease (PID), and possible infertility.

Threatened Miscarriage   Threatened miscarriage is defined according to how many weeks along the pregnancy is.

Have: immediate medical help and total bed rest

Try: tea or tinctures, diluted in water:

Dioscerea villosa (wild yam root)	1 ounce
Anemone pulsatilla (pasque flower herb)	2 ounces
Passiflora incarnata (passionflower herb)	2 ounces
Viburnum opulus (cramp bark)	3 ounces
Viburnum prunifolium (black haw bark)	3 ounces
*Cimicifuga racemosa** (black cohosh root)	1 ounce

*Only use black cohosh during the last six weeks of pregnancy.

Decoct 1 ounce of herb mixture in 3 cups of water; take ½ cup every half-hour, or as needed.

Remember, labor is initiated by the baby, not when the uterus or the mom is "ready." No herb can keep an embryo in that is not going to be compatible with life. These herbs, plus supportive nursing care, may prevent a miscarriage.

After Miscarriage   To return normal tone to the uterus, balance hormones quickly, and promote emotional equilibrium:

Angelica archangelica (angelica root)	3 ounces
Symphytum officinale (comfrey leaf)	1 ounce
Achillea millefolium (yarrow flower, herb)	1 ounce
Vitex agnus-castus (chasteberry seed)	1 ounce
Hypericum perforatum (St. Johnswort herb)	2 ounces
Cimicifuga racemosa (black cohosh root)	2 ounces

Because the woman is no longer pregnant, this may be taken as tincture, one teaspoon diluted in water three to four times a day for a minimum of thirty days.

As an alternative, this may be taken as a tea. Combine roots and seeds in one container, herbs and flowers in a second. Decoct ½ ounce of roots and seeds in 3½ cups of water for 20 minutes; turn off heat and add ½ ounce of herbs and flowers. Replace cover; infuse for 10–15 minutes. Strain; drink 3 cups a day for two months or less, as needed. The two-step process in one saucepan can be done in larger batches to save time. Stored in the refrigerator, a batch lasts three days.

This is such a difficult experience. No herbs can replace grieving, resting, counseling, love. Continue to see your primary care provider. Flower remedies may help; please see Resources.

Prevention of Miscarriage (with Previous History) Have: sound nutrition, meditation, system tonics (if one body system is significantly weaker than the whole woman is, see "Tonics for Use During Pregnancy," earlier in this chapter).

Visualize how you have changed since the last experience. Your past is not your potential. We are not doomed to repeat history. There are changes you can make with every bite of food, with every thought you allow into your mind, and every word out of your mouth.

Avoid: heavy lifting, taking on extra stress, skipping meals

Try:

Viburnum prunifolium (black haw bark)	2 ounces
Rubus idaeus (raspberry leaf)	4 ounces
Mitchella repens (partridgeberry herb)	½ ounce
Leonurus cardiaca (motherwort leaf)	¼ ounce

Infuse 2 teaspoons per cup for 20 minutes, then strain; take 1 cup two to four times day, as needed, throughout pregnancy. Though motherwort is bitter and potentially stimulating to peristalsis, this small amount in combination with relaxing astringents is helpful to nerves in liver health.

During Early Labor Have: raspberry leaf tea already made into ice, broken up into chips to suck on when your mouth feels dry, instead of drinking lots of liquid

Try: doing nothing; less is more; a basically healthy woman does not need much herbal help with labor

If a very pregnant woman wants to drink herbal tea to make life more pleasant at this stage, the following may be taken liberally over one to two days:

Rubus idaeus (raspberry leaf)	1 ounce
Mitchella repens (partridgeberry herb)	1 ounce
Matricaria recutita (chamomile flowers)	2 ounces
Passiflora incarnata (passionflower herb)	3 ounces

Steep 2 ounces of herbal mixture in 3 cups of water for fifteen to twenty-five minutes; drink ½–2 cups of tea.

Long or Stalled Labor Have: a nap, a walk around the room—for some women, a walk outside for an hour

Stalled labor is often due to exhaustion; it describes normal labor that has stopped progressing as expected. If pathological problems have been ruled out, relaxation is most important.

Try: time alone with your partner, nipple stimulation, gentle lovemaking without intercourse.

Tinctures are more convenient than tea for therapeutic use at this stage. Make the following labor tincture in advance (see Chapter 2: Herbal Preparation); if you use tea (infusion + decoction), make it fresh daily or refrigerate it for up to eighteen hours before discarding. Note: This herbal formula may lower a woman's blood pressure. This amount of herb formula is usually within the safe range, though a sensitive woman may feel dizzy if she stands too quickly. Since long labor accompanies lack of energy, one precaution would be to eat something before rising from a completely horizontal position. Dizziness might just be a symptom of long labor.

Caulophyllum thalictroides* (blue cohosh root)	1 ounce
Cimicifuga racemosa (black cohosh root)	1 ounce
Mitchella repens (partridgeberry herb)	2 ounces
Rubus idaeus (raspberry leaf)	2 ounces
Cinnamomum spp. (cinnamon bark)	¼ ounce

*Use blue cohosh only during the last four weeks of pregnancy.

Take ½ teaspoon of this formula diluted in 1 cup of warm water every fifteen to forty-five minutes, or as needed. Alternatively, a woman may prefer to sip this slowly throughout her waking hours for energy.

Goldenseal is oxytocic (stimulates uterine contractions); although its effects are not always safe, it is often used or recommended by others. It is not safe to use except during the last days of pregnancy, and then only to stimulate stalled labor under the supervision of a health care provider familiar with stages of delivery. Tincture or glycerin extract of goldenseal can be given separately in 15-drop doses every twenty minutes as needed (one #00 capsule is the equivalent, but it takes longer to have an effect, therefore is less predictable and less recommended here).

Painful Labor/Contractions   Have: partner help focus concentration, coach with breathing techniques, massage if the woman *wants* it (she may want no one near her)

Try: tincture of two antispasmodic herbs:

Cimicifuga racemosa* (black cohosh bark)	1 ounce
Dioscorea villosa (wild yam root)	1 ounce

*Use black cohosh only during the last six weeks of pregnancy; otherwise omit it.

Take ½ teaspoon of combined tincture diluted in water every twenty minutes, or as needed.

As a tea, this can be useful if made ahead of time. Decoct 1 ounce of dry herb mixture in 2 cups of water for fifteen to twenty minutes. Strain the tea, and drink ½–1 cup every hour, or as needed.

If tincture or tea is not effective, take up to 1 ounce of tincture divided in 1-teaspoon doses diluted in water, using any one or more of: skullcap, passionflower, valerian. This is usually a short-term problem.

To Calm and Help "Ground" Those in Attendance   Have: Rescue Remedy, a flower essence combination for tension; Royal Jelly, a high protein bee product for energy; easily digested food nearby but in another room. Both products are available at most herb shops or natural food stores.

Try: herb tea. This could be a big pot of the formula described in "During Early Labor" elsewhere in this section, or 1–2 teaspoons per cup of any one or more of the following: catnip, chamomile, lemon balm, linden.

Expelling the Placenta   Have: the baby at your breast, gentle massage of the uterus (lower abdominal massage), nipple stimulation. It should come out on its own. Raspberry leaf taken during labor also helps.

Try: one to three cups of angelica and/or basil tea if the placenta is retained. Alternatively, use 1 teaspoon of tincture (if both herbs are used, equal parts), diluted in a little water every six hours, up to three times. If that doesn't work, try a glass of wine or a dose of goldenseal (1 teaspoon tincture or glycerin extract, or 1 #00 capsule with a glass of water).

After the birth, it is normal to have approximately three to four days of red discharge, then pink discharge, until it changes from pink to white by the ninth day. If there is still red discharge, there may be retained material; see a health care provider.

After Birth Is Over   To tone and involute the uterus (return womb to its new "normal" position) more easily:

Vitex agnus-castus (chasteberry seed)	1 ounce
Melissa officinalis (lemon balm herb)	1 ounce
Crataegus spp. (hawthorn berry, leaf, flower)	2 ounces
Foeniculum vulgare (fennel seed)	1 ounce

Infuse 1–2 teaspoons of dry herbal mixture per cup of water for twenty minutes; drink one cup three times a day for two weeks.

Disinfecting the Cord   Have: for external use, one of the following: goldenseal powder, comfrey leaf tea or tincture, propolis tincture, myrrh and calendula tinctures (equal parts). Sprinkle powder on externally. Alternatively, use herb tea/ tincture on a clean, soft cloth as a disinfecting compress for five to ten minutes twice a day to speed healing.

Avoid: cotton balls, because wisps left behind may cause minor infection or irritation

Breast-Feeding   Have: a list of good reasons for breast-feeding (see below), just in case you or your friends need reassurance about your choice.

Try: La Leche League (in the telephone directory) or nurses for information and much-needed support for the new mother whose level of fatigue and frustration mount if the baby isn't eating; it is not always easy to get a newborn to latch on.

Sometimes babies want to suckle for comfort more than for food value, so a mother may need safe herbal nervines to help keep her calm and centered with the inevitable sleep-deprivation, toddlers, partner, and other daily demands that will attempt to divide her attention during the first weeks of frequent, long feeds.

See "Galactagogues" in "Safe Herbs for Pregnancy and Lactation," earlier in this chapter; use standard preparations of any one or more.

Positive Reasons for Breast-Feeding:

- great bonding and establishment of healthy future relationship
- better immunity for baby, especially against allergies
- helps prevent breast cancer in mother
- associated with reduced risk of SIDS (Sudden Infant Death Syndrome), among other cofactors
- mother's milk protein is genetically tolerated by baby, so no known case of reactions
- keeps baby's guts sterile until appropriate flora develop
- reduces dental caries and cravings for sugar in children
- prevents sterilization/expense/hassle of formula and bottle routine in the middle of the night

Reasons Not to Breast Feed:

- inability of baby to thrive on mother's milk
- breast cancer
- AIDS
- psychological disturbances in mother

To Increase Milk   Have: oatmeal (if it appeals to the mother), seeds, nuts, whole grains, peas, and sprouted seeds and legumes (alfalfa, others). These provide B-vitamins, plant proteins, fatty acids, and mildly estrogenic plant compounds to nourish a new mother and provide rich milk for the baby.

Avoid: dairy products, garlic, onions, hot peppers. These tend to create gas or colic for the baby.

Try: 1 ounce per pint (standard preparation) of one or more of the following galactogogues: milk thistle (after delivery), vervain (after delivery), goat's rue, vitex, nettles (large amounts okay after delivery). Fennel, dill, and anise are especially useful if the baby is colicky.

To decrease excess milk production, drink sage leaf tea (standard preparation); it is safe for a woman to drink while she is breast-feeding but most helpful at weaning in order to reduce excess milk production.

Post-Partum Depression   For one in ten new mothers, the joy of having a baby is fraught with challenges, as elation gives way within a matter of days to post-partum depression (PPD). This is characterized by frequent crying, extreme feelings of being unable to cope, or even fear of hurting the baby. This may lead to a confused neglect, in the hope that avoiding the baby will keep it safe. PPD can occur any time in the first year of a baby's life, and women who have it often feel embarrassed and guilty. Shame can be made worse by family, friends, and societal conditioning, which may pressure a woman into feeling she can't "do it right," or that "self-discipline" will cure her of depression.

Sudden changes take place in hormone levels after a woman delivers a baby. LH, estrogen, and progesterone levels rise throughout pregnancy—up to fifty times higher than before pregnancy—over a matter of months. These levels drop within hours after delivery, when the level of estrogen remains low, with very little progesterone. During this resting phase, the pituitary response to GnRH (gonadotropin releasing hormone) is low, and the ovarian response to LH is also low.

It is difficult to predict which women will experience PPD, as almost half of new mothers experience some mild "baby blues." Risk factors for PPD include a positive family history, PPD after a previous birth, personal history of mood illness, low thyroid, sleep disturbance, being raised in an alcoholic or dysfunctional family, an unusually fussy or needy baby, delivering a premature or compromised baby, discord in the primary relationship, severe PMS prior to pregnancy, ambivalence toward becoming a mother, isolation from family and friends, lack of emotional or financial support, and lack of self-care (eating well, regular exercise, interest in life).

Diagnosis requires individual assessment with lab evaluations, while treatment may include family and personal counseling, education, and support groups. Many women resist antidepressant drugs during this time, and prefer to try natural, less aggressive remedies.

It's important for a new mother to feel safe expressing less-than-ideal emotional responses to having a new baby. An emotional support network (local new mothers group) that lasts for the baby's first year can be very helpful.

Herbs with a supportive hormonal and nutritive effect include chasteberry (*Vitex agnus-castus*), raspberry leaf (*Rubus idaeus*), nettle (*Urtica spp.*), motherwort (*Leonurus cardiaca*), and mild bitter digestive tonics, such as dandelion leaf and root (*Taraxacum officinale*). Use standard preparations of any one or more of these. See your health care provider if there is no change in one to three weeks.

Herbs with Limited Use in Pregnancy

Aloe vera is used externally as a demulcent vulnerary for burns.

Bearberry (*uva ursi*) is used to treat cystitis before trying antibiotics only if five days use of more gentle osmotic diuretics such as corn silk, echinacea, and marshmallow have not worked (see corn silk or "Cystitis," earlier in this section).

Black cohosh is not a tonic for long-term use (usually during last six weeks). It is an antispasmodic used with cramp bark and black haw against threatened miscarriage (see "Threatened Miscarriage," earlier in this section). It is also given in the last two to four weeks of term to treat false labor pains, cramping, or nervousness; its relaxing nervine properties may help a woman save energy for delivery. The dose is ½ teaspoon of tincture diluted in a small amount of water, herb tea, or juice, taken every hour as needed.

Blue cohosh root is not a tonic for long-term use (usually during last four weeks). It acts as an antispasmodic, oxytoxic, and a tonic to the womb and fallopian tubes. Use fifteen drops of tincture in water or under the tongue after labor has begun—*if* labor is prolonged and *if* the mother is fatigued—for exhaustion and pain. Small doses are also helpful for expelling the placenta; for this use, it combines well with angelica root and basil herb (see "Long or Stalled Labor" and "Expelling the Placenta" earlier in this section).

Chasteberry is used after delivery when it promotes involution and milk production, but it is not indicated during pregnancy.

Comfrey has been used by pregnant women in times past with no apparent ill effects. The herb world still debates the safety of this herb rich in one constituent (pyrolizidine alkaloids) that may be harmful due to the sensitivity of growing embryonic tissues in pregnant women. Err on the side of caution. Use comfrey externally as the wonderful demulcent vulnerary that it is for superficial tears and wounds, and as an excellent herb oil to massage into the vagina and entire perineum, stretching the perineum in order to avoid episiotomies. For directions on use, see "Preventing Tears," earlier in this section.

Goldenseal is oxytocic (stimulates uterine contractions, helps bring on labor). It is not given internally any time during pregnancy before labor. A dose of one-half teaspoon in water every half-hour is sometimes still used by midwives instead of castor oil for slowed labor. It is not safe or recommended to use without a midwife or other care provider's supervision. Glycerin extracts (tinctures without alcohol) are easier to take, and are commercially available. For alternatives, please see "Long or Stalled Labor," earlier in this section.

Herbs to Avoid During Pregnancy

During the first and second trimesters, avoid the following (also see "Herbs with Limited Use in Pregnancy," earlier in this section):

> black cohosh - *Cimicifuga racemosa* (use during the last six weeks only if needed)
>
> blue cohosh - *Caulophyllum thalictroides* (use during the last four weeks only if needed)
>
> comfrey - *Symphytum officinale* (externally only)
>
> cotton root bark - *Gossypium spp.*
>
> goldenseal - *Hydrastis canadensis*
>
> suma - *Pfaffia paniculata*
>
> yellow dock - *Rumex crispus* (½ cup tea in combination with bulk fiber or carminatives is okay to relieve constipation, but may be stimulating to lower intestines early in pregnancy)

Throughout the pregnancy avoid:

aconite - *Aconitum napellus*

aloe - *Aloe vera* (externally only)

American ginseng - *Panax quinquefolium*

American mandrake - *Podophyllum peltatum, P. spp.*

American mistletoe - *Phoradendron flavescens*

arnica - *Arnica montana* (except homeopathically or externally)

astragaulus - *Astragalus membranaceus*

barberry - *Berberis vulgaris, Berberis spp.*

bloodroot - *Sanguinaria canadensis*

bogbean - *Menyanthes trifoliata*

broom - *Cytisus scoparius*

bryony - *Bryonia dioica*

celery seed - *Apium graveolens*

chaparral - *Larrea spp.*

coltsfoot - *Tussilago farfara*

comfrey - *Symphytum officinale*

elecampane - *Inula helenium*

ma huang - *Ephedra sinensis*

false hellebore - *Veratrum viride*

fenugreek - *Trigonella foenum-graecum*

feverfew - *Chrysanthemum parthenium*

gentian - *Gentiana lutea*

ginkgo - *Ginkgo biloba*

ginseng - *Panax ginseng*

greater celandine - *Chelidonium majus*

hops - *Humulus lupulus*

horehound - *Marrubium vulgare*

hyssop - *Hyssopus officinalis*

ipecac - *Cephaelis ipecacuanha*

Jamaican dogwood - *Piscidia erythrina*

jimsonweed - *Datura stramonium*

juniper - *Juniperus communis*

lad's love - *Artemisia abrotanum*

licorice - *Glycyrrhiza glabra*

lobelia - *Lobelia inflata*

lomatium - *Lomatium dissectum*

male fern - *Dryopteris felix-mas*

meadow saffron - *Colchicum autumnale*

mistletoe - *Viscum album*

mugwort - *Artemisia vulgare*

nasturtium - *Tropaeolum officinale*

Oregon grape root - *Berberis aquifolium*, synonym: *Mahonia aquifolium*

pennyroyal - *Mentha pulegium*

Peruvian bark - *Cinchona spp.*

pleurisy root - *Asclepias tuberosa*

poke root - *Phytolacca decandra*

poppy - *Papaver somniferum*

quassia - *Picrasma excelsa*

red sage - *Salvia officinalis var. purpurea*

rue - *Ruta graveolens*

sage - *Salvia officinalis* (Note: Small amounts in cooking or mouthwashes are fine; safe to consume during lactation, even helpful for drying up excess milk when baby is ready to be weaned.)

sassafras - *Sassafras albidum*

saw palmetto - *Serenoa serrulata*

senna - *Cassia senna*

Siberian ginseng - *Eleutherococcus senticosus*

tansy - *Tanacetum vulgare*

thuja - *Thuja occidentalis*

thyme - *Thymus vulgaris* (Note: Small amounts in cooking or mouthwashes are fine.)

vervain - *Verbena officinalis* (fine after delivery)

wild carrot - *Daucus carota*

wild indigo - *Baptisia tinctoria*

wormseed - *Chenopodium ambrosioides*

wormwood - *Artemisia absinthium*

yellow jasmine - *Gelsemium sempervirens*

yucca - *Yucca baccata*

Nutrition

Depression is more closely linked to nutritional habits than has previously been acknowledged by the conventional medical view. Drinking more than four to five cups of coffee a day is linked to depression, as are low levels of vitamin B_6 and B-complex, which affect nerve stability.

Some studies show that depressed people are more likely to have low levels of folic acid, which in turn may lower their serotonin production. Serotonin is derived from tryptophan. As a supplement this was banned, probably without due cause after a single batch of contaminated tryptophan was identified. Tryptophan is available in the seeds of evening primrose (*Oenothera biennis*), though amounts vary with different preparations. The recommended dose after delivery of the baby is two capsules (500 milligrams each) twice a day for six to eight weeks.

Other deficiencies associated with depression are calcium, magnesium, potassium, and iron.

Two other findings associated with depression are extremes of dietary fat (either too high or too low) and food allergies. In the case of food allergies, an underlying physical problem, such as *Giardia*, has been mistakenly diagnosed at least once as depression. This might be because symptoms of pain, food sensitivities, and fatigue may lead to, or mimic, depression.

Begin with a varied, whole-food diet with several colors of plants (organic local fruit in season, leafy dark greens, sprouted seeds and legumes, yellow and orange carrots or squash, red beets and bell peppers, brown rice, whole grains).

Eliminate caffeine, refined foods, and potential sources of low-grade irritation from food sensitivities or allergies. Common dietary allergens are: dairy products (yes, all kinds), eggs, soy, wheat, and food additives (preservatives, colorings, flavorings).

Supplements

Supplements and herbs may not be metabolized in the low-stomach acid often found with depressed people. Increase the stomach acid with digestive bitter tonics, such as radicchio and artichoke salads at the beginning of main meals. Garnish vegetables and salads with lemon juice and garlic rather than heated butter or heavy, commercial salad dressings.

Pre-natal supplements with folic acid are best determined for each mother-to-be by her care provider. Consider increasing foods high in vitamins. Vitamins and minerals extract well into therapeutic infusions, but are not as reliable for nourishment in the form of tinctures.

- Foods with B vitamins: asparagus, leafy green vegetables, and whole grains (rice, millet, amaranth, quinoa (pronounced KEEN-wah), and buckwheat)

- Herbs with one or more nutrients in the B complex: nettles, raspberry fruit and leaf, rose hips, parsley, slippery elm, and red clover
- Foods with vitamin C: raw broccoli florets, baked potatoes, horseradish, rose hips, peaches, and citrus
- Herbs with C complex: raspberry fruit, rose hips, dandelion greens, chickweed, red clover, and parsley
- Foods with iron: include raisins, prunes, figs, and blackstrap molasses (1–2 teaspoons a day)
- Herbs with iron salts or which may raise hemoglobin are: kelp, yellow dock root, nettles, milk thistle seed
- Herbs with magnesium are: oat straw, nettles, red clover, raspberry leaf, and chickweed
- Potassium: bananas
- Herbs with potassium: red clover and nettles
- Essential fatty acids: *freshly ground* flax seed, evening primrose seed, and purslane

Other Points

If you cannot hold urine when you laugh, sneeze, strain, or jump up and down, then you need to do Kegel exercises and "elevator rides." These two exercises cost no money, require no classes, and are best started some months before delivery, as early in pregnancy as practical or even before conception. Even a few weeks of these before birth makes a difference. Like yoga, the more consistently and the more slowly these are done, the better the effects.

Kegels (usually pronounced KAY-gels, to rhyme with "bagels") help the mother's reproductive muscle tone. Kegels are very safe. These strengthen the muscles that make up the pelvic "floor." Our pelvis is like a big basin or fruit bowl, with openings at the bottom that we control through muscle tone. These muscles have the most fascinating names: the *pubococcygeus* muscles are a pair that stretch from the pubic bone in front to the tail bone in back, like a mirror image with one on each side of the central urethra, the vaginal opening, and anus. Another pair are the *coccygeus* muscles that connect the tailbone in back to the bones at the right and left sides of the pelvic basin. These two pairs of muscles are symmetrical, and look like flower parts or butterfly wings holding your insides inside. They are reinforced by external pelvic muscles and structures. The *perineum,* a band that stretches from the center out to the right and left connecting to the sides of the pelvic basin like an arched rainbow, lies between your vaginal opening and the anus. This perineal skin can be massaged with an herbal oil to make it more elastic and stretchy to avoid tearing or episiotomy (see "Preventing Tears and Episiotomies," earlier in this chapter).

Kegels also help to bring good blood flow and muscle tone to the perineum. There are two sphincters in the pelvic floor. We have one muscle sphincter around the urethra and vagina, and another around the anus. A sphincter is like a donut of muscle—if you clench the sphincter around the urethra and vagina, you can stop urine passing. To feel this muscle, try an experiment. The next time you are sitting on the toilet to pass urine, tighten your muscles to stop the stream of urine. Let it go. Stop it again. You have just done two Kegels. Now that you know from the experiment which muscles to "feel," repeat this tightening and letting go when you are not passing urine. Repeat and count them in groups of ten or fifteen groups of four, or whatever you are comfortable doing.

Kegels can be done anywhere at anytime: standing at the counter making dinner, sitting in your car at a stoplight, or waiting in lines. Women can do Kegels whether or not they are pregnant for any reason, including better orgasms. It is a simple contraction and release. These can be done during intercourse if desired. Not only will these exercises improve muscle tone to prevent or lessen complications of pregnancy (from hemorrhoids to miscarriage), doing them now will speed the recovery of vaginal tone after delivery.

The second exercise—called elevator rides—is simple, too. Tighten the sphincter muscles at the outermost surface of skin around the anus and vagina. Count to five, and release. Tighten again; as you count to five this time, contract the muscles around your birth canal higher and higher, like an elevator going up. Hold as tightly at the "top" as you can do in comfort for a count of two. And then, slowly, SLOWLY, SLOWLY come back down, feeling where there is great control and where there may be a little less control. Work on making the elevator ride smooth up and down, imagining your baby's eventual ride down being as smooth under your own control as you can possibly make it. Although the actual birth may feel like it is on its own unstoppable course, having done these for weeks or months beforehand will make all the difference.

For the emotional challenges that are inevitable during pregnancy and family life, don't forget about song, goofing off, serious prayer, and flower essences for part or all of the family when any one of you is under serious stress.

16

Herbal Baby Care

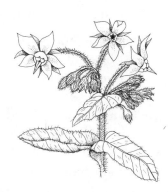

Whenever possible, the natural therapist prefers to treat the baby's problems with herbs filtered through the mother's breast milk. Therefore, the herbs for babies discussed in this chapter are given as preparations for the mother to drink, unless otherwise stated. The protective nature of mother's milk screens any foreign chemicals from the baby. As a result, the baby's later tolerance to foods is promoted because the liver and immune system are not challenged with strange proteins before the baby is mature enough to take food and drink by mouth (six months to two years).

Herbalists recognize that breast-feeding isn't always possible. Many conventional and alternative formulas are available; each has pros and cons, so ask your local midwife, nurse-practitioner, or other health care provider for information about the method that best suits your baby's needs.

Jaundice   Have: sunlight, breast-feeding

Try: for the mother, one cup twice a day of dandelion and nettle tea (equal parts, standard preparation). If the baby must be bottle fed, try a sterile infusion at one-third strength in a bottle for three to seven days.

Diaper Rash   Have: baby naked after the bath if possible; add ¼ cup apple cider vinegar to the rinse cycle of diapers

Avoid: commercial talc

Try: replacing talc with the herbal baby powder formula that follows; massaging the baby with: three drops each of lavender and chamomile essential oils diluted in one ounce of green olive, sesame, or grape seed oil (let absorb before diapering or clothing)

Herbal Formula for Baby

comfrey leaf powder	2 ounces
calendula flower powder	½ ounce
white or green cosmetic clay	⅛ cup
cornstarch or arrowroot powder	⅛ cup

Optional: Add six drops total of chamomile and/or lavender essential oils per batch of powder. Sift well; store in a brown paper bag for a few hours before using. Does not require refrigeration. Use as needed.

Teething Pain   Give: zwieback or melba toast, something pleasant to chew on, homeopathic chamomile (use as directed on package label). Homeopathy works as well as herbal medicine, if prescribed appropriately. If this doesn't work, herbs may have a more immediate effect.

Try: a drop of blue chamomile essential oil massaged by a clean finger on the spot. Having the baby suck on a clean cloth dipped in chamomile tea may help, too.

Some babies respond well to the use of cold to numb the gums; small ice cube chips made of strong chamomile tea can be wrapped in a clean cloth for baby to chew on.

One mother told me that she didn't have time to do anything but put chamomile flowers in a clean cloth, dampen it with hot water, and let her baby gnaw on that. The inflamed gums stopped looking so red, the baby stopped crying, and, after his nap, the tooth was peeping through the gums without further problems—for that tooth, anyway.

Eye Care   Have: a diagnosis first; if a minor eye problem is self-limiting, it may be soothed and its healing may be hastened with the following formula. For a problem passed within a household or circle of small children, this will speed the body's ability to fight off infection. It may also rinse out minor irritations such as dust, animal dander, or sand. For any eye condition that gets worse after a day or two, see your health care provider.

Euphrasia officinalis (eyebright herb)	¼ ounce
Glycyrrhiza glabra (licorice root)	¼ ounce

Make this as *100% sterile* tea; if a dishwasher or other method of sterilization is not available, immerse all utensils in rapidly boiling water for twenty minutes. Pour 3 ounces of water that has boiled rapidly over herb mixture. Steep, covered, for fifteen to twenty minutes; add 1–2 drops tincture of benzoin or chamomile essential oil as a preservative and additional anti-inflammatory. Shake oil and water together well, because they don't mix.

Store in a sealed container in the refrigerator for no more than two days. To use as wash or compress, check the temperature in your own eye before using it as a wash for a baby's eyes. Using an eyedropper, drop five to twenty drops into the inner corner of the eye, tilting the baby's head so that it flows to the outer corner of the eye as the baby blinks. Repeat every few minutes (or as child allows), twice a day. After two days discard the unused portion and sterilize the container and eyedropper. If needed, make another batch.

Infants' Infections   Have: a thermometer to gauge whether herbs are working or not

Avoid: refined sugar or excess honey to make herbs taste better, because these feed bacteria and fungi and depress immune-system function. Also avoid cold draughts and late nights (see "Insomnia" in Chapter 15).

Try: for the mother, whether she is breast-feeding or not, up to three cups per day of echinacea decoction, or four half-teaspoon doses of tincture daily for three to ten days

For babies who can take a bottle, use 12 teaspoons of echinacea tincture in 6–8 ounces of water every two to four hours as needed, or ¾ cup of decoction diluted with ¾ cup of water. For high fevers or listlessness, see your health care provider.

As an alternative to echinacea, use ¼ ounce of vervain infusion (standard preparation). Vervain is safe during lactation, but possibly too stimulating during pregnancy. It promotes healthy amounts of breast milk and digestive juices. It also tastes pretty bitter, so add to equal parts by weight of licorice root for taste.

Externally for infections (for example, on an uncircumcised penis), follow basic good hygiene and adequate air-drying, and apply 1 teaspoon myrrh propolis tincture dipped in ¼ cup water.

Colic   Have: dill, fennel, and ginger in the mother's diet. Have a quiet, warm place for nursing, and a relaxed attitude even though both mother and baby may be exhausted

Avoid: laxatives, all dairy products (at least for a week to assess), chocolate, peanut butter, refined sugar, and white flour in the mother's diet. If that doesn't work, try avoiding vegetables in the Brassica family and others known to cause intestinal gas for babies who are breast-fed: cabbage, Brussels sprouts, broccoli, turnips, radishes, kale, collards, cauliflower, garlic, hot peppers, and hot spices.

Try: goat's milk if the baby is bottle-fed, or weak (but sterile!) herb teas. Use chamomile, catnip, and/or anise: ½ ounce to one pint steeped ten minutes; strain and pour 4 ounces with added water into the baby's bottle. Repeat every two to eight hours for one to two days, or as needed.

Paroxysmal Fussing   Have: faith; defined as a three-month colic, this is worsened by fatigue and an annoyed family

Avoid: drugging the baby with sedatives

Try: for the mother, 1 teaspoon of motherwort tincture three times a day. For mother and baby, use 1 ounce of herb to 1 pint of water (standard preparation) of any one or more of these teas to taste: chamomile, passionflower, skullcap. Take one-half to two cups as frequently as needed. If needed for more than three days, be generous with added herbs for flavor. Choose from lemon balm, hibiscus flower, cinnamon bark, mint, and aniseed.

Give the rest of the household or family a thermos full of the same tea and a day's outing somewhere.

Oral Thrush   Have: a little garlic in the mother's diet if it does not cause intestinal upset for mother or child. You can mash garlic and mix a few drops of this into a teaspoon of unsweetened yogurt, and apply it to the raw patches of this fungal infection.

Homemade or live yogurt with helpful bacteria can be used on its own, dabbed onto raw patches in the mouth. See Chapter 19: Candida for further information.

Avoid: refined sugar in both the mother's and child's diet

Try: rinsing the baby's mouth and mother's nipples with diluted calendula tincture (¼ tablespoon per 2 ounces water) or calendula tea (standard preparation) before and after every feeding.

Alternatively, soak one teaspoon of psyllium seeds for an hour or more (they can sit covered overnight); dab the slimy gel on raw patches of red tissue in the mouth to soothe (it is safe for the baby to swallow).

Cradle Cap   Have: a massage for baby's scalp using herbal oil (comfrey or calendula, but no essential oils). Herbal oil may be purchased or made at home (see Chapter 2: Herbal Preparation). A thin film of this oil may be left on overnight to make it easier to gently remove loose flakes in the morning (don't pull off pieces of skin that are not ready); reapply. Between massages, gently clean the scalp by dampening it with a tea of witch hazel (1 ounce, decocted 10 minutes and strained; not distilled extract from a drugstore); let tea cool to the same temperature as the baby's scalp, and apply it with a soft cloth two to several times daily for one to four days.

Internally and externally, give violet flower and leaf infusions (standard preparations, in a bottle or via mother's milk). Johnny-jump ups and sweet violets (not other ornamental pansies) can be grown easily at home, and the fresh flowers and leaves (made into a standard infusion) double as a hair rinse for the baby and a tea for mother and/or baby.

Mild Fevers Have: a sense of balance about whether this needs medical treatment or love. Babies and growing children can get fevers from hearing loud crashes or sensing parental discord, so don't assume the worst—just pay attention. In a study of more than one hundred children with all the signs of an upper-respiratory infection (fever, runny nose, coughs, tiredness, some vomiting), only two had bacteria that could be cultured. The rest showed symptoms that would have caused their pediatricians to prescribe antibiotics. Check with a health professional if a diagnosis is needed, but meanwhile there are safe things to do at home.

The fever should respond to treatment within a few hours, after a night's sleep, or in two days; otherwise, see your health care provider just to be sure.

Use sponge baths and soaking in "tea baths" made of any one or two (not all at once) of these fever-reducing herbs (double strength but otherwise standard infusions): catnip, fennel, elder, willow bark, meadowsweet, echinacea. Give the baby extra attention.

Avoid: sugary or oily treats, pizzas, and mucus-forming foods (dairy, oatmeal, excess bread) for mother or baby, especially dairy products

Try: for the mother, two teaspoons of echinacea tincture diluted in water each day while breast-feeding; babies can take echinacea tea or glycerin tincture (up to three half-teaspoons diluted in water daily, for ten to twelve days)

Crying Have: a sense of these quick descriptions to distinguish when to get outside help or what your baby wants. The loudest cries are often about comfort and security.

Hunger is not usually the first cry or the loudest, but comes second after desires for cuddling, comfort, and security have been satisfied. Hunger cries are not resolved for long by giving comfort; that's one way new parents come to recognize the baby's only way of communicating.

Shrill cries may signal emergencies, including *intussusception,* in which the baby's intestines are trying to learn peristalsis but instead of contracting in rhythmic downward waves, the guts get stuck and "telescope" one segment into the next—most painfully, with a sudden, astonished cry. This and other painful conditions need medical attention.

Frightened cries may accompany emotional changes in those near a baby, or mishaps that do not result in harm, when calm comfort is the best medicine; interpretation may be difficult, so there is always the option of calling a care provider when in doubt.

Croupy cries may result from a throat or lung infection, including laryngitis. A grunt is associated with pneumonia.

A croak is associated with Down's syndrome children, while a whimper usually comes from older children. *Cri du chat,* or "cat's cry," is a howl associated with an uncommon hereditary disorder too complex to be covered here; see your health care provider.

Baby Insomnia   Have: a thermometer to check for temperature (rooms or sleep wear may be too hot for their active little metabolisms). Keep their changing room at about 72°F, like the temperature of a newborn, but allow them to feel colder air during sleep or at times other than changing. Also bathe the baby in relaxing teas (formulas follow), in a baby tub or with a parent in the bathtub.

Avoid: baby's possible discomfort from itching, including from acrylics or wool, irritation, wet diapers, or twisted clothing. Check with your health care provider for causes of respiratory problems: a cold, blocked nose, adenoids. Check for other types of discomfort: thread worms (give ¼ clove garlic, chopped and disguised in 1 teaspoon honey), pain, strange noises, or unfamiliar beds. Infections such as worms from pets or other children respond well to reduced sugars, juice, and honey, although a little honey with garlic is fine for babies taking food by mouth (but not newborns).

Try: an herb tea that is soothing and calming, such as the formula below. Catnip, an ingredient in the formula, does not have the same effects in humans—even tiny ones—that it does in cats. It is a mild, relaxing nervine tonic, good for fussiness, indigestion, and fevers.

Matricaria recutita (chamomile flowers)	1 ounce
Nepeta cataria (catnip herb)	1 ounce
Trifolium pratense (red clover flowers)	1 ounce

Steep 1 ounce of herbal mixture per pint of water for fifteen minutes; strain tea and give ½–1 cup in a bottle as needed.

You can also make a baby herb pillow, and leave it under the baby's sleeping pillow or near the bedding:

Rosa canina (rose petals—no hard flower buds)	1 ounce
Lavandula spp. (lavender flowers)	1 ounce
Matricaria recutita (chamomile flowers—no stems)	1 ounce
Nepeta cataria (catnip herb)	1 ounce
Rubus idaeus (raspberry leaf)	1 ounce

Don't add mugwort, often found in adult dream pillows. Babies are close enough to the place of dreams; they need restful sleep, not excited adventures of the subconscious. Mix the herbs and place them in a cotton drawstring bag or sew a closed bag of soft flannel. These herb pillows can be drooled on or chewed safely, but a tightly closed bag avoids accidental choking on loose pieces of herb.

Baby Lotion   For dry skin or massage lotion, use the following:

avocado, walnut, or grape seed oil	¾ cup
distilled or floral water (rose, orange flower)	¾ cup
beeswax	½ ounce

Melt oils and wax together over the lowest possible heat; cool so that the mixture will still pour. Put water in a blender running at the highest speed; slowly dribble the oil/wax mixture into the water until it blends, like making homemade mayonnaise. Add fifteen drops total of essential oils as a preservative, using one (or two at the most) of the following: lavender, chamomile, orange, rose. It takes a few tries to get perfect lotion. Store in a clean plastic squeeze bottle or wide-mouth glass jar with a close-fitting lid. Note that rubber-lined canning lids for mason jars will be ruined in a few months by contact with oils.

PART FIVE

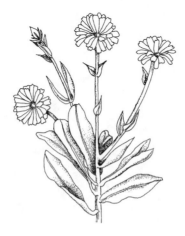

Infections

17

Urinary Tract Infections

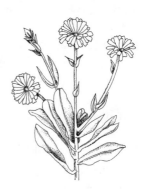

Definition

The linings of the bladder and other urinary tract structures are designed to hold wastes, occasional sugars and germs, and the warmth necessary for germs to grow. These urinary tract linings have evolved to secrete antiseptic substances. In health, this keeps things under control.

We are not meant to be sterile creatures. In health, only our urine and the bladder itself are sterile. When we give a urine sample for diagnosis, we avoid contamination with the normal microbes of the external genitalia by letting a little of the stream of urine pass, washing out superficial bacteria at the exit. The midstream flow is collected and analyzed; a bacterial count of more than 100,000 creatures per ml (milliliters) of urine, or even lower in some cases, means there is an infection of the lower urinary tract. This urinary tract infection is abbreviated "UTI."

Symptoms and Signs

Microbes irritate the bladder and cause frequent urination, fever, fatigue, and other symptoms. There is a feeling of urgency, when it seems that one cannot wait to urinate but little comes out. This is accompanied by frequency because the irritation of the bladder and urinary tract structures signals the nerves that the bladder must be emptied. Most distressing, perhaps, is *dysuria,* or painful urination, due to muscle spasms and burning as urine passes inflamed linings. Frequent urination may lead to getting up during the night to void the bladder, so fatigue is common after only a few days.

As with any infection, there may be fever, chills, and pain in the lower back, abdomen, or one side. If pain is severe, there may be nausea and vomiting. Sensitive women and children may have abdominal discomfort and diarrhea, even without fever. These symptoms may respond to bed rest, eating lightly, and clearing the infection, but if fever rises above 102.5 degrees F, or if you feel worse after one to two days, see your health care provider.

Cause

When stress, antibiotics, hormone imbalance (the birth control pill, hormone replacement during menopause), or other factors of illness upset internal control over common urinary infections, simply increasing the "river" will help. In a larger stream of urine, the contents move out of the body more swiftly, and bacteria and other organisms are diluted in a larger volume of water. Common bacteria that cause lower UTIs are *E. coli*, *Proteus*, *Enterobacter*, *Pseudomonas*, and *Klebsiella*.

These irritants are often neutralized by herb constituents or natural defenses in the increased flow of urine. The body's self-healing mechanisms regain their normal function after the worst of the invasion is handled this way.

Less common causes of chronic UTIs include kidney stones and structural blockages.

Many urinary tract infections start as untreated or inadequately treated vaginal infections. Some parts of the body, such as the bloodstream, are alkaline under healthy conditions. Some places like to be acidic; two examples are the vagina and urinary tract. An acid pH keeps out microbes that would grow in these locations if they were alkaline. Such normally acidic areas may become alkaline if a woman is stressed, or when acid-secreting friendly bacteria are wiped out by antibiotics.

There are other ways in which these usually acidic locations become alkaline, including washing genitalia with soap instead of plain water, using "feminine hygiene" products, overdouching, and poor nutrition. Nutritional triggers to alkalinity include eating too much sugar or red meat, or drinking too little water.

Conventional Medical Care

The conventional treatment is a wide array of antibiotics such as Amoxicillin, but these frequently cause candidiasis of the genitalia (see Chapter 19), reproductive tract, or other systems, with the possibility of an ascending infection leading to cystitis (bladder infection) or even potentially dangerous infections of the kidneys. Antibiotics may or may not work; their use is debated. If the right antibiotic for the infecting organism is used, the urine should be clear of bacteria in three days, with a follow-up urine test in two weeks. Because common microbes become resistant to short-term use of antibiotics, it is important to complete any antibiotic therapy started.

There is a caution, however. Infections can start simply but if they are ignored, or treated inadequately with either herbs or antibiotics, infection can spread upward and do serious damage.

Another conventional treatment for resistant UTIs with kidney problems is dilation of the urethra to prevent blockage of urine.

Herbal Treatment

The holistic objective is to reduce inappropriate numbers of bugs and beasts (pathogenic organisms), improve the host's tissue-resistance to damage from the infection, relax muscles that may be in spasm, and improve natural immune-system response, thereby preventing reinfection. When women increase their consumption of water, certain juices (such as unsweetened cranberry) and antimicrobial diuretic herb teas, the excretion allows the urinary system to flush out most problem-causing microorganisms and return to its normal sterile condition.

The purpose of the following herbal formula is to return the acid-alkaline balance of the urinary tract to normal so that the body's defenses can take over from there. Taking cranberry juice, bearberry (uva-ursi) tea, or other herbs that work this way (also vitamin C) to acidify helps the body to cleanse and normalize itself.

Herbal Formula I

Arctostaphylos uva-ursi (uva-ursi leaf)	4 ounces
Althaea officinalis (marshmallow root, leaf)	3 ounces
Achillea millefolium (yarrow flower)	2 ounces
Cinnamomum spp. (cinnamon bark)	1 ounce, or to taste

Follow standard directions for preparation and dosage. Drink a minimum of two cups, up to a maximum of five cups, a day for ten days. It is important to keep drinking one to two cups per day for a full week to ten days after all symptoms have cleared.

Note: During pregnancy, omit yarrow; see safe herbs for cystitis in Chapter 16: Pregnancy.

The active disinfecting constituent in Herbal Formula I is the *arbutin* in *Arcto-staphylos uva-ursi* (uva-ursi, bearberry), which is stronger than the active ingredient in cranberry juice. This only gets activated as a urinary disinfectant in the kidney tubules, the ureters, inside the bladder, and down the urethra. This "activation on site" of the herb where it is needed works well even when the pH environment inside the urinary tract is alkaline—the way the urinary tract is likely to be if infected.

If painful muscle spasms, especially on urination, are a significant problem, add to Herbal Formula I:

Viburnum opulus (cramp bark)	2–3 ounces
Zingiber officinalis (ginger root)	¼ ounce

If pain on urination (dysuria) is the dominant symptom, add:

Zea mays (corn silk)	2 ounces
Althaea officinalis (marshmallow root)	2 ounces
Echinacea spp. (echinacea root, any species)	4 ounces
Equisetum arvense (horsetail herb)	1 ounce

These can be used as a standard tea (best), 1 ounce to 3 cups of water, one cup three times a day, or tincture (dilute 1–2 teaspoons in one 8-ounce glass of water, three times a day). See Chapter 2: Herbal Preparation if more information is needed.

Symptoms may improve within two to three days, but these formulas are safe for continual use for up to four weeks (except during pregnancy; see Chapter 16). If no improvement is seen within forty-eight hours, you may want to see a health practitioner for a follow-up.

For interstitial cystitis, use:

Herbal Formula II

Serenoa serrulata (saw palmetto berries)	3 ounces
Equisetum arvense (horsetail herb)	1 ounce
Achillea millefolium (yarrow herb)	2 ounces
Hypericum perforatum (St. Johnswort herb)	2 ounces
Passiflora incarnata (passionflower herb)	2 ounces

Follow standard preparations and dosage, ½ cup of tea four times a day, for a minimum of eight weeks.

If there is tenderness over the groin or abdomen and a fever above 101 degrees F, herbal treatment used alone must work fully within three to five days. Otherwise, stubborn infections can lead to more serious problems; these are avoided with adequate treatment. To determine whether alternative remedies have worked fully, get a clean-catch urine sample tested. The herbs work, but there are no guarantees from a book to a reader, so the reader's health must be assured by another person such as a health care provider who can analyze urine.

Herbs are strong antimicrobials, especially active in the pH of the urine or in biological "compartments" like the bladder. Herbs can be taken along with conventional medical care, and in fact discourage the growth of opportunistic infections following drug treatment.

External Herbal Therapies

Hot sitz baths help increase circulation and help immune-system cells in the bloodstream to get to the areas where the UTIs are located.

One option is to follow a sitz bath with an external massage of pain-relieving, antimicrobial essential oils:

sandalwood essential oil	5 drops
ginger essential oil	5 drops
geranium essential oil	5 drops
almond oil	½ ounce

Mix five drops each in one-half ounce of warm almond oil; massage for five to ten minutes over the lower back and abdomen.

Nutrition

Avoid refined sugar and refined products; follow a basic whole-food diet and, in recurrent or severe cases, a three-day cleansing fast.

If possible, eat nasturtium leaves and flowers (*Tropaeolum majus*)—a sharp and delicious disinfectant—in fresh salads: up to 1 ounce of fresh material per day. Growing your own keeps you in fresh supply. They are beautiful and low maintenance, and they grow like a weed, even in urban apartments.

Four or more glasses of natural, unsweetened cranberry juice (not commercial, corn syrup- or glucose-sweetened) is recommended daily. The ideal is to eat lightly the first day or so, taking cranberry juice on an empty stomach, about four hours after eating. Advertisements for concentrated pills of the active constituent in cranberries are misleading, in my opinion, because cranberry plant acids and glycosides don't do much good in a capsule for women who also need to increase the amount of fluid flushing through their system.

Unsweetened or naturally sweetened (white grape) fruit juices, or vegetable juices (beet, celery) are effective, especially diluted by half with good-quality spring water, or taken over the course of a day in addition to eight glasses of water. Herbal tea or tinctures may also be diluted in water.

Other Points

Part of the holistic treatment is abstinence from sexual intercourse (with penetration) until the woman is completely well.

18

Vaginitis

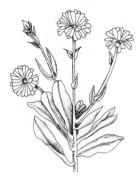

Definition

Vaginitis simply means an inflamed vagina, though there is not always an inflammatory response. Many women use this term to mean any number of conditions in which there is irritation of the vagina. The proper medical term for vaginitis due to bacteria is *bacterial vaginosis* (BV). The term includes the vulva and other external genitalia, not just the vaginal canal. Irritation in one part of the female genital region easily triggers inflammation in surrounding parts. Irritation happens at every age for a variety of reasons. Vaginitis responds well to herbs and integrated medicine.

Cause

Vaginitis isn't always caused by an infection, though various microbes are common causes. The most frequent infecting organism for nonspecific vaginitis is *Gardnerella*. *Gardnerella vaginitis* is an STD that is sometimes called *hemophilus;* this gram-negative bacteria is a *facultative anaerobe,* which means that it hates oxygen. Bacteria are classed by the way they take up stains in the lab, either gram-positive or gram-negative. Males with *Gardnerella* show no signs or symptoms. Two other common organisms causing vaginitis are the yeast *Candida,* and the protozoa *Trichomonas.* Vaginitis can also be caused by three other venereal infections: gonorrhea, genital warts, or herpes virus Type II.

When an infecting organism is not the cause, the inflammation of vaginal linings may be due to hormonal imbalance. This occurs at many stages of a woman's reproductive life. It is also common when our bodies adjust to a naturally lower level of ovarian estrogen during menopause (see Chapter 23).

Vaginitis can be caused by factors as diverse as stress, nutritional imbalance, or inadvertently leaving in a tampon, diaphragm, or other foreign object.

Problems originating in the external genitalia that may lead to inflammation of the vagina include pubic lice or crabs, wounds that develop secondary infections, or chemical causes including reactions to feminine hygiene sprays, scented or colored toilet tissue, detergents, and hot tub chemicals.

Vaginal irritation is a good way to bring a woman's loving attention to her body's most tender gateway, where imbalances, subtle or severe, are made obvious.

Symptoms and Signs

A Quick Look at Vaginal Symptoms

Color	Feels Like	Smells Like	Other	Possible Cause	What to Do
clear	stretchy, rubbery	normal		ovulation, sexual stimulation	up to you
milky	creamy	normal		pre-ovulation	nothing
white	sticky	normal		post-ovulation, taking the birth control pill	maybe nothing
brown	watery, sticky	almost normal		end of menses, spotting	nothing
white	watery, like buttermilk, creamy	normal or foul, fishy	itchy, possible fever	bacterial vaginitis, *Gardnerella?*	treat, monitor
white	flecks, like curds	yeasty, foul	itchy	*Candida*	treat
yellow	smooth or frothy	foul	itchy, may be red dots on cervix, possible fever	*Trichomonas?*	treat, monitor; see medical practitioner
yellow or green	thick mucus	normal or foul	cramps, dysuria, possible fever	PID, possibly gonorrhea (even with no discharge)	see medical practitioner

Conventional Medical Care

Flagyl is used, along with antibiotics such as Clindamycin, in pill form and vaginal ointments and gels. If *Gardnerella* is cultured from a woman who has no symptoms, no treatment is recommended. If sexual partners are male, it is uncertain if treatment is necessary. Flagyl is not considered safe during the first trimester of pregnancy; Clindamycin and Amoxicillin are often used. If these drugs are taken, it is important to finish the course even if symptoms disappear quickly.

Herbal Treatment

The holistic objective is to restore normal flora and tone to the mucosa. This can best be done with the herbal actions of anti-inflammatories, astringents, and demulcents. Antimicrobial herbs are often used to prevent or treat vaginitis, even if it is not caused by infection, because inflammation makes a woman more vulnerable to secondary infection. Herbs that prevent secondary infection also heal and soothe, such as *Plantago spp.* (plantain leaf), *Calendula officinalis* (calendula flowers), and *Glycyrrhiza glabra* (licorice root).

The following herbal treatment allows inappropriate microbes to be removed with few of the side effects of antibiotics, antifungals, or other drugs. Opportunistic organisms such as candida are reduced by many of the herbs in the formulas found in this section, but please refer to Chapter 19. Herbal formulas can help the body's own defenses to reduce these problem organisms to levels considered nonpathogenic by the immune system (*not* masking subclinical infection, but rather existing in a natural balance).

Herbal Formula

Plantago major lanceolata or	
P. lanceolata, P. spp. (plantain leaf)	2 ounces
Cimicifuga racemosa (black cohosh root)	2 ounces
Anemone pulsatilla (pasque flower herb)	3 ounces
Levisticum ligusticum (lovage herb)	1 ounce
Glycyrrhiza glabra (licorice root)	¾ ounce
Thymus vulgaris (thyme herb)	¾ ounce

Prepare a standard infusion and take the standard dose for two weeks, for up to three months. Alternatively, combine these tinctures or extracts and take 1 teaspoon diluted in water after meals three times a day.

During pregnancy, leave out black cohosh, licorice, and thyme; replace with echinacea and nutritional use of garlic, plus local (external) use of marjoram in the second or third trimester only, using the directions detailed in "External Herbal Therapies," below.

This compound can be expected to bring results in one to two weeks, but can be taken safely for up to four weeks, at which time reassessment is recommended. It is always wise to continue taking smaller maintenance doses of herbal formulas for another week or two after symptoms have cleared.

For more deep-seated infections, add:

Echinacea spp. (purple coneflower root)	2 ounces
Calendula officinalis (calendula flowers)	½ ounce

External Herbal Therapies

If vaginitis is due to dryness or vaginal thinning during menopause, see Chapter 23, or use:

External Herbal Formula I

Thymus vulgaris (thyme herb)	2 ounces
Symphytum officinale (comfrey root)	1 ounce

Steep 1 ounce of the mixture in one cup of boiled water for twenty minutes. Strain well and use one to two times a day, depending on the severity of symptoms. This makes an excellent external wash for the labia, vagina, and external genital tissues. Allow one to two weeks for results.

If vaginitis is due to *Gardnerella*, use externally:

External Herbal Formula II

Commiphora mol-mol (myrrh resin)	1 ounce
Calendula officinalis (calendula flower)	1 ounce
Quercus alba (white oak bark)	1 ounce

These are best used as tinctures, combined in equal parts. Use one teaspoon of each to a pint of water, used externally as a douche, penis soak, or wash for both partners, done every day for three to seven days.

External Formula III isn't herbal, and over-douching isn't healthy, but the organism of *Gardnerella* does respond well to this while the internal Herbal Formula (page 195) is taken. The use of hydrogen peroxide in the vagina repeatedly introduces oxygen to the oxygen-hating *Gardnerella*. This is astringent (toning) and disinfecting, and allows a natural change in the vaginal environment to one that supports healthy vaginal flora.

External Formula III

hydrogen peroxide (3%)	1 tablespoon
water (distilled or sterilized)	1 cup

Douche with this mixture once or twice a day for one week, then repeat less frequently as needed perhaps every three days for an additional two weeks. Following a retest to see if the organism is clear, continue the internal Herbal Formula for another week to ten days. If there is no response in a total of two to three weeks, please see your health care provider to reassess the vaginitis.

If vaginitis is due to candida, please see Chapter 19.

If vaginitis is not clearly due to one particular microorganism or cause, follow the internal herbal recommendations for up to six weeks along with the following all-purpose, external douche. The herbs have an anti-inflammatory, antimicrobial, and astringent action on the vaginal walls—not drying, but toning and moistening. See a practitioner to follow up, whether or not symptoms clear up.

External Herbal Formula IV

Achillea millefolium (yarrow flower)	1 ounce
Plantago spp. (plantain leaf)	3 ounces
Calendula officinalis (calendula flower)	2 ounces
marjoram essential oil	¼ ounce

Steep 1 ounce of a mixture of the first three ingredients in one pint of boiling water, covered, for 45 minutes or until cooled to a comfortable temperature for vaginal use. Strain tea; then add 4 drops of marjoram essential oil per fluid ounce of herb tea. For example, add 32 drops in 8 ounces of herb tea. Mix well. Douche without rinsing afterward, every day for one to two weeks.

Nutrition

Especially when vaginitis is associated with chronic yeast, avoid sugar, refined flour products, and processed foods. Even excessive honey, maple syrup, and fruit juices may delay the full effects of an herbal approach. As with most conditions, nutrients from a whole food diet are recommended because they accelerate the removal of symptoms and may prevent recurrences. Add foods rich in B-complex (whole grains), vitamin E, and essential fatty acids to the diet (avocado, flax seed, wheat germ).

For vaginitis associated with menopause, several foods such as sprouted seeds with essential fatty acids, soy, vegetables with vitamin E (avocado), and nutritive roots help vaginal tone (please see "Nutrition" in Chapter 23).

Supplements

Daily recommendations include:

>   vitamin C: 1–5 grams
>   vitamin A: 10,000 IU for 6 weeks
>   zinc: 15 milligrams for 1–3 weeks

19

Candida

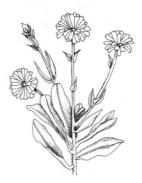

Definition

When people speak of candida, they may be speaking of any of at least four related phenomena. Candida is both a yeast and a fungus, depending on when you examine it. The organism was formerly called *Monilia*. An infection with this is called *Candidiasis* (formerly *Moniliasis*). The infection commonly occurs in the vagina, and that's what most women are referring to when they say they have candida. But the term "candida" may also mean an overgrowth of the yeast or fungus in someone's intestines, or even in the entire system of a person, resulting in the condition called "systemic candidiasis." Many people believe they have systemic candida, when in fact, this is a life-threatening condition found only in severely immunosuppressed people such as those with AIDS or cancer. Only vaginal, oral, or digestive candidiasis can be treated with herbs. So candida is a yeast, a fungus, a local infection of the external genitalia (in either gender), or an infection of the digestive tract or the whole system of a person.

Vaginal yeast is a common complaint. It is common because of the abuse of powerful antibiotics and symptom treatments of opportunistic yeast by advertised "cures." Candida is not handled well by the drugs once prescribed by doctors—now sold over the counter at pharmacies. The recurrence of yeast infections after using these drugs is high. Despite advertising campaigns by drug companies, the availability of these compounds over the counter is not a great breakthrough in women's liberty, because these conventional antifungals kill more good bacteria than candida, leaving women more vulnerable to repeat infection—and, of course, repeat purchases. Many strains of candida are now thought to be resistant, so inadequate symptom suppression and rate of reinfection are also high.

Commercials pushing antifungal suppositories are not the worst: Women have been exposed over the years to the message that "clean" women spray chemicals up inside themselves. Feminine hygiene sprays may lead to or worsen infections, inflammation, and unhealthy beliefs about the human body—oh, yes, and the apparent need to buy *more* deodorant spray. Feminine hygiene products are worse than useless. Cheap perfumed chemicals do not cover up odor, but they do aggravate the body's attempt to self-clean.

In health, women's vaginal secretions do not smell "bad." Women may have a strong aroma, especially when one is down close to the source. Women with an offensive odor have a health imbalance. In health, the liver, kidneys, lungs, skin, and intestinal tract divide up the chores of elimination.

All these natural functions may be improved with herbs. Alterative tonics help when sweat glands and skin pores are basically healthy but the organs of elimination are working flat-out to eliminate metabolites from a woman's intake of meat, alcohol, and drugs (including some prescription drugs). Candida and other organisms have characteristic odors. Bad smells are a way to warn us not to spread a possible organism, or irritate raw linings with impatient intercourse.

Symptoms and Signs

Candida, the books say, looks like cottage cheese. I never saw cottage cheese that looked like that. Candida is usually more like a collection of bluish-white to cream-colored clumps seen on the labia and inside the vagina. There may be a few small isolated patches, or it may look like a membrane spread over a large section. If you pull away the clumps, little stringy threads can be seen—these are from fungal "feet" buried in the tissue. Where the clumps are removed, the tissue underneath is red and raw-looking. It may be swollen as well as inflamed, or it may look eroded below the surface of the surrounding normal tissue. On the mucous membrane of the vagina, this candida can be yellow—an indication of heat or inflammation. It smells sour, like old milk products. It makes sex and urination painful.

On the outer skin, candida looks scaly, red, and raised. There may be a rash with little red raised spots, with or without discharge. In women with large breasts, candida occurs underneath where the skin stays moist and warm. It can also appear in the folds of the groin, armpits, and fingers. On the nails of hands or feet, the nail bed (skin under and surrounding the nail) becomes a discolored red to purplish, especially apparent when the weather gets cold. Left untreated, candida growth can progress until discharge pushes the nail away from the flesh. In Great Britain, this condition is called "barmaid's hands" because barmaids are likely to have their hands wet, washing glasses in soapy water or holding foamy mugs of yeasty beer. A fungus can overgrow on any surface that stays warm and wet, especially without a healthy immune system.

In the mouth and throat, candida may occur on the tongue or other surfaces, causing a burning sensation during swallowing or eating. Soothing herbs for the rawness (*Althaea officinalis*—marshmallow root) mix well with the antifungal plant extracts (see "Herbal Treatment" later in this chapter) to make a mouthwash; you swish it around and spit it out, then drink a cup.

Yeast infection of the external genitalia occurs in men, too, though possibly without symptoms other than a reddened glans of the penis or plaques below the foreskin. Not all women show that they are carrying candida, either.

Candida is such a normal part of the microbial mix on the planet that even healthy babies may get candida growing in their mouths, called "thrush." It is a sign that the baby needs rest, fluids, and a change of foods, or the mother needs to improve her diet while she's breast-feeding. It is common, but it's not healthy or normal if it is severe or recurrent. A tea of calendula flowers may be swabbed inside the baby's mouth, with the edge of a very clean, soft cloth, dipped in the tea. Repeat a few times a day until all the white curds are cleared out of the baby's mouth. If a breast-feeding baby has oral thrush, mother should swab her nipple area and baby's mouth before and after feeding with the calendula flower tea to minimize the spread. If the baby drinks from a bottle, check how sterilization between feedings is going. Leave all dairy out of the diet. Babies don't need cow's calcium to grow if they receive breast milk, plant seed "milks" such as soy or sunflower, or any form of green, leafy vegetables. Leave any sugar or refined foods out of the diet. Remember, most babies need these minor exposures to microbes to develop immune resistance against further infection. Antibiotics and antifungals may or may not work with infants, but even if they do the bad news is they short-circuit the baby's ability to flex its own immune muscles. Use antibiotics only if thrush is seriously threatening your baby's health. Pregnant women with vaginal candida may pass it to infants during birth. Prevention (resting, eating well) are safer than treatments later.

The signs of systemic candida are serious. The infection, which is rare in people who can still go about their regular daily lives, comes with chills and a high fever, or one that spikes rapidly; the blood pressure drops and there is faintness, dizziness, and fatigue. People who truly have systemic candida need to lie down because of extreme weakness. Rest is essential in their holistic treatment which almost always includes intravenous antifungal antibiotic drugs. To be certain, common infections with candida are not "systemic" though they may be chronic. Systemic candida can travel and start overgrowing in different locations, giving different clues. In the lungs it may cause coughing, possibly including coughing up sputum mixed with a little blood (from blood vessels broken by coughing). In the digestive tract, candida can cause bloating, especially with certain foods such as sugar, excess starch (grains), alcohol, and other potentially irritating substances. Kidney signs include pain on the sides of the torso and problems with urination, especially cloudy or bad-smelling urine. There may also be headaches, rigidity of the muscles supporting the head, or seizures. Heart signs include heart murmurs, chest pain, or emboli. An *embolism* is a blood clot or other piece of tissue that is loose in the blood stream where it may lodge in a blood vessel, causing blockage and damage. In the eye, there may be painful inflammation, blurring of vision, or even discharge.

With all of these symptoms, a hundred other causes might be responsible. It is easy to assume candida but the best care comes from determining the cause with your health care provider.

Cause

Most cases of candida involve *Candida albicans* (*alba* means "white," like the discharge this causes). Several other less common *Candida* species exist. These are a part of the normal flora of the human gastrointestinal tract from the mouth all the way down, as well as part of the normal flora on the skin and vaginal lining. In health, the other flora keep candida growth limited so that it doesn't cause much harm. We always "have" candida. We have an *infection* when some body change allows it to grow unchecked.

The first point to establish is that the organisms are not out to kill you, and they do not require a militaristic attitude about taking every known antifungal. They don't *know* you don't want them to multiply; *you* gave them the perfect environment. How?

Yeasts love sugar—they thrive on it. Increased blood sugar levels can result from dietary choices, excessive alcohol consumption, or endocrine disorders, including diabetes. Eating sugary foods or filling up on bread instead of fruit, vegetables, and other whole foods leads to high blood sugar.

Lowered resistance causes candida overgrowth. Other diseases, lack of sleep, and taking corticosteroids and other immunosuppressive drugs, such as those used to treat cancer, are all known to trigger this infection.

Use of antibiotics, especially the broad-spectrum ones such as tetracycline, is notorious for wiping out healthy flora, leading to candida overgrowth.

Irritation of any one area of tissue, if repeated steadily enough, can cause candida. This includes vomiting due to bulimia or alcoholism, IV (intravenous) therapy or drug abuse, and ill-fitting dentures. Elders with dentures already have a risk for each of the cofactors causing candida if their nutrition is limited; for instance, inexpensive, easily digested white bread. They may have a lowered resistance due to the use of antibiotics for frequent infections or other health challenges due to age.

Candida loves warm, moist environments with little or no circulation: tight nylon underpants, one-piece cat-suits, and spandex sportswear. Women can wear these clothes if they balance doing so with relaxing in loose clothes of natural fibers.

Poor hygiene is implicated as a cause of candida overgrowth. Plain water without soap is best. Washing thoroughly means rinsing away visible clumps of yeast with water. Not even "natural" soaps are needed. Soaps are all based on the saponins that cut through grease so that water can rinse away oil and dirt. Leave other protective bacteria and vaginal enzymes undisturbed by soap, as they are part of your natural immunity for this entryway to the body. We are self-cleaning, not intrinsically dirty. Dry carefully to avoid re-irritating sensitive patches that are trying to heal after washing.

Another common cause related to hygiene is not wiping from front to back; the bacteria of the anal skin can upset the vaginal bacteria and cause infections. It may seem too obvious to state, but this is still a common cause of introducing bacteria from the rectal area to the vagina.

Systemic candidiasis has been erroneously linked in the popular view to Epstein-Barr Virus, Chronic Fatigue Syndrome, Attention Deficit Disorder, hypoglycemia (low blood sugar), and chronic degenerative disease. This opportunistic infection is a concern in diabetics and HIV-positive people, since they are particularly sensitive to high levels of sugar in the blood and to immune-system dysfunction, both of which trigger candida overgrowth. In multi-system illness, systemic candidiasis is related to inflammatory conditions, particularly "leaky gut" syndrome, itself a source of debate.

Conventional Medical Care

The conventional view of candidiasis is that it is not passed back and forth from sexual contact. It supposedly starts and recurs only from spreading candida from one's own normal skin or intestinal flora to places with compromised immunity, where it seizes the opportunity to flourish. It seems from clinical experience that when immunity is low for any of the known factors (from blood-sugar level to fatigue), candida can be spread by contact with someone else's normal skin or intestinal flora.

Many health care providers presume that reinfection can come from an untreated partner if a woman tests clear, takes no new courses of antibiotics, remains healthy for a few months, finally feels "safe" to have intercourse with the same untreated partner she had before, and has a recurrence. To be fair, the cause of reinfection may not always be so obvious. The immune-system response to the presence of foreign proteins *other* than the partner's candida may trigger an inflammation. This could cause a woman's candida to flare up.

The conventional treatments for candida are Nystatin or ketaconazole, Diflucan or fluconazole, or other standard antifungals (several come in cream or pill form, and all get mixed reviews from candida sufferers). The fluconazole drugs kill off candida in its mycelial phase more successfully than antifungal herbs, and so are necessary especially for immunosuppressed people with mucosal candidiasis. Multisystem candidiasis cannot be treated without drugs. Gentian violet is still used on fingernails and toes, but the residual stain made it go out of fashion for treating skin fungal infections (this product is not made from the gentian herb; it is an antifungal chemical dye, methyl-rosaniline chloride).

The conventional treatment for systemic candida is intravenous antifungals and antibiotics. Remember, systemic spread of candida internally is not identical to chronic vaginal candida.

Herbal Treatment

The natural way to help women's bodies fight this common microbe is with liquids, rest, and a different choice of foods. Herbs are usually taken as liquids (teas, tinctures diluted in water, and fresh vegetables on our plates). The herbs listed in the formulas below and recommended in the "Nutrition" section of this chapter are disinfecting, but many of them are also gentle relaxers, taking the edge off symptoms until the cause is cleared up. This way, we can get on with our lives, but without suppressing the real cause of the candida.

The holistic objective with a systemic candida infection is to reduce inappropriate numbers of this normal flora to a nonpathogenic level while reducing causative cofactors, such as stress, inappropriate diet, and immune-system imbalance, including antibiotic use. Long-term management by diabetics and others at risk can prevent this organism from causing destructive changes without impairing a person's immunity. This approach revolves around regular eating and wise food choices.

An herbal blend for maintenance may be changed over time, as long as it always contains an antifungal herb such as *Calendula spp.* (calendula flowers) or *Juglans nigra* (black walnut hulls), a nutritive nonspecific tonic such as *Urtica dioica* (nettle leaf) or *Taraxacum officinale* (dandelion root and leaf), a nervine tonic such as *Nepeta cataria* (catnip), and an herb to stabilize blood sugar such as *Verbena officinalis* (vervain herb), *Achillea millefolium* (yarrow flower), or *Oplopanax horridum* (devil's club root bark, *not* devil's claw). This is not a prescription, but an outline of suggestions to cover attitude, nutritional state, blood-sugar stability, and immunity. Herbal antifungals usually have one or more of these additional properties, rather than relying on a single chemical constituent for its "antifungal" power.

The holistic treatment using herbs may be directed toward a local vaginal infection, and it may need to be directed to a systemic infection. If vaginal yeast reoccurs, a serum and/or stool test for systemic yeast is recommended. A blood test for antibodies to candida indicates the presence of an immune-system response, pointing to excess candida growth if there are definite lesions and symptoms. But even this does not diagnose systemic candidiasis. Another test is used to identify budding cells of candida from swabs or scrapings of tissues lining the vagina, skin, mouth, or other tissues. In systemic candida it is necessary to diagnose by a culture from blood or tissue that would not show this common organism's presence in a state of health.

Candida infects not only our tissues but our thoughts, until we see it everywhere. Early in my practice, I saw a woman who had all the symptoms listed in best-selling books on the subject of candida. She had been on the prescribed anti-candida diet for months. Yet she swore she still had vaginal and systemic candida, and she wanted herbs to help finish the job. There was no visible discharge on clinical examination, and I requested lab tests.

I had doubts about her self-diagnosis after taking her case history, since her symptoms of sensitive vaginal membranes and food sensitivity could be explained in other ways, but I didn't want to be disrespectful of her strong assertion that she had candida. Doctors had been unhelpful. She "knew" that her self-diagnosis was correct from reading the books, so she refused to see another doctor or pay for lab tests.

I found myself in a legal and ethical bind. The law states that, since this country does not recognize my European degree, I cannot make the diagnosis I was trained to make, or I'll be jailed for practicing medicine without a physician's license. Besides, it is a holistic ideal to honor the patient's view of her own health. My oath is to serve to the best of my ability. After consideration, I gave her the herbs to treat candida and had her come back in for follow-up soon afterward.

I should have known better when the antifungal herbs still had no effect on the "candida." But maybe she was right, the popular books were right, and this was a tough case. I knew she was under stress from relationship changes. We used stronger antifungal herb extracts. No improvement. She was extremely disciplined about following a stricter diet than I would have recommended, considering her overall health and the minor but persistent degree of vaginal discomfort she was experiencing. I wanted her to be in charge of these treatment decisions after she heard my recommendations and reviewed her options. I asked colleagues including doctors of oriental medicine and allopathy for insights, and tried everything. The herbal medicine I used could have wiped out the yeast cultures of an entire bread-baking Zen community.

Finally I convinced her to get the lab tests. There was not a shred of a yeast survivor on her vaginal tissue culture or from her stool. No blood signs of infection. The doctors she saw for lab interpretation said they had never seen such a whistle-clean, healthy vagina. Every immune-system cell was present in the right numbers, and in a state of peaceful readiness.

She was mad at *me* because she still had the same symptoms she associated with candida. Many intelligent people treat their candida like a precious burden they carry around with them—out to dinner, into bed, everywhere. We hear that we are supposed to listen to the wisdom of our bodies, but this business of trusting oneself is tricky. Her "illness" wasn't yeast but oversensitivity (from an extremely limited diet), motivated by subtle self-punishment and guilt for what she perceived as sexual "mistakes." The happy ending is that we talked. I gave her the mildest relaxing nervine herbs, and soon she was perfectly healthy again.

This is not to say that candida is all in a person's imagination, or that a woman who does not respond to treatment does not want to be well. When tests indicate that this opportunistic infection is present, it may indeed be difficult to clear up. Without judgment, I can only report that people with candida overgrowth need more than an herbal antifungal or repeated courses of antibiotics to achieve homeostasis. Effective treatment is influenced by other factors. Herbs have an edge over some drugs as antifungal therapy because, while the antifungal action of herbs is strong, these plants are rounded out with other healing properties such as improving digestion, reducing bloating or gas, and relaxing tension that often worsens candida.

Some therapists have observed a relationship between the way this opportunistic infection takes over the tissues and the way women with chronic candida tend to let opportunists run their lives. Physiologically, candida grows only when immune-system barriers are weak. If a person with candida also has a passive personality, a holistic herbal approach is to improve physiological immunity with psychosocial defenses. There is beauty in knowing how and when to be passive. Candidiasis is one example of too much of a good thing becoming a negative state, feeding disease.

Holistic health practitioners believe that candida gets passed back and forth so easily between sexual partners that abstinence makes herbal treatment work faster and more completely. Of course, all partners must be treated successfully. Let your partner know that abstinence is not a punishment; it just makes healing easier. Anyone can get an infection; getting candida carries no shame. It's how you treat the infection that shows how you feel about sickness and, in this case, sex. Honor the temple of the body with temporary abstinence during treatment if what you want is good sex.

Holistic treatment takes into account the fact that so much tension builds up when a couple can't have sex, because one partner is "infected," that stress is laid on the one person who needs less stress in order to self-heal. In reality, sex invites individuals to join in partnership. Sex means that the health of one is not separate from the other. Sex allows us to share intimate joy as well as responsibility for the health of the sexual couple.

It doesn't hurt for the partner who has no symptoms or is "well" to drink the same herbs for infection, too. With such a persistent organism as candida, genuine healing is best shared by both halves of the whole. In any case, any sexual partner should be treated, whether or not she or he has symptoms, especially if the partner is an uncircumcised male. Yeasts can hide under the foreskin or on the shaft without giving symptoms to the man. Hygiene and shared herbal self-help can help to dissolve tension (penis soaks are amusing to describe or do). Medicine does not have to be dignified or solemn to be effective. If women drink herbs and cautiously douche, what do men do? See "Penis Soaks" under "External Herbal Therapies" in Chapter 21: Trichomonas.

Herbal antifungals are preferred over repeated use of conventional antifungals because after initial use of fluconazole for example, they have fewer side effects. The body knows how to take antifungal substances as they are found in nature and use them or lose them in normal elimination. The more we tinker with antifungal molecules, the less able the body's chemistry is to handle the stronger chemicals; hence, unexpected reactions and side effects occur.

Pau d'arco, the first herb in the following formula, is an antifungal plant from South America, pronounced "pow-DAR-ko." Because this herb is often placed with similar-looking substitutes in commerce, ask for evidence that your resource has the genuine herb. If your questions can't by answered satisfactorily, use this formula without pau d'arco. Black walnut hulls are astringent and antifungal. These require decoction, while the other herbs in the same formula are added after simmering to preserve their medicinal volatile oils and other constituents. Licorice is a soothing anti-inflammatory, and stimulates digestion, elimination, and immunity.

Herbal Formula I

Tabebuia impetiginosa (pau d'arco bark)	3 ounces
Juglans nigra (black walnut hulls)	3 ounces

Mix these two together, and store in a separate container.

Althaea officinalis (marshmallow root)	2 ounces
Nepeta cataria (catnip herb)	2 ounces
Calendula officinalis (calendula flower)	2 ounces
Glycyrrhiza glabra (licorice root)	1–3 ounces, to taste

As always, this is a conservative dose per day of licorice, but if licorice is contraindicated because of water retention or high blood pressure, leave it out or replace it with an equal amount, to taste, of *Illicium verum* (star anise seed pods).

This is a two-part recipe, but it can be prepared in one saucepan. Simmer ½ ounce of the first mixture (equal parts of black walnut hulls and pau d'arco bark) in 3 cups of water for fifteen minutes, on medium-low heat, covered.

Turn off the heat, stir in ½ ounce of the second mixture (marshmallow root, etc.), and let these steep together for ten more minutes. Strain and drink one-half cup before and one-half cup after every meal. This is not enough liquid to over-dilute digestive juices, and it will even help assimilation of nutrients from meals.

Extra half-cups may be taken whenever symptoms appear, up to eight half-cups per day for as long as six months. However, if the symptoms show no signs of improvement in one month, check your herbs or check your diagnosis.

If systemic candida and intestinal gas are an additional problem, add:

Mentha piperita (peppermint leaf)	3 ounces
or	
Elettaria cardamomum (cardamom seeds)	3 ounces

Adjust to your taste. After two days, you will feel better and the herb tea will taste better to you. Don't discontinue sooner than two weeks.

If bowel pain is a factor, add:

Valeriana officinalis (valerian root)	1 ounce
Dioscorea villosa (wild yam root)	1 ounce

If stress is a predominant cofactor for candida flare-ups, add:

Scutellaria lateriflora (skullcap herb)	1 ounce
Passiflora incarnata (passionflower herb)	1 ounce

External Herbal Therapies

Marjoram is especially good as a simple antifungal. Besides enjoying it in cooking, which is helpful but not strong enough to rely on, it can be used as a douche to clear candida vaginally. The easiest and mildest herbal formula for vaginal application follows:

External Herbal Formula I

Aloe vera gel	4 ounces
marjoram essential oil	25 drops

Mix the two ingredients together and store in a container with a tight-fitting lid; keep in the refrigerator. If you are mixing one day's application at a time, use 2 drops of marjoram oil to 1 tablespoon of aloe gel (since the aloe gel is cold from the refrigerator, you might want to let it warm up a bit before applying). Apply gel liberally to coat the inside surfaces of the labia, morning and night; wear a panty liner. Aloe is soothing and vulnerary (heals surface tears, burns, and wounds), while marjoram essential oil reduces yeast in the moist environment of the vagina and external genitalia. This can be used for men externally, as well. Lavender or ti tree essential oil can replace marjoram essential oil.

In stubborn cases, antifungal therapy can be as simple as inserting a peeled clove of garlic vaginally. You don't even have to like eating it to get the benefit. Peel the stiff, papery coverings off carefully. Leave the thin membrane on the garlic or wrap the clove in one thin layer of gauze so that the garlic juice isn't too strong on direct contact with painful, inflamed mucous membranes. Dipping the garlic clove in olive oil makes it easier for some women to insert. Leave in overnight for eight hours of local antifungal effects; this can be repeated nightly, but is not usually needed after two to five nights unless there is chronic candida (long-term or recurrent vaginal infection). Garlic cloves are small enough to slip out the next morning when bearing down, as when urinating or moving the bowels.

Another way to use garlic vaginally for candida is to place a square of thin gauze around a peeled clove of garlic, then tie a piece of dental floss around the gauze where it is gathered in a bunch. Insert in the vagina, leaving the "tail" of dental floss hanging down so that the gauze and garlic can be retrieved later. Without this, garlic cloves may dissolve inside overnight because of our metabolic processes and body heat. There is no harm if the garlic dissolves, but some women prefer to remove the used clove.

Once a patient called in the middle of the night: "I can't find it. Should I go to the emergency room and *tell them?!*" If it's just the garlic that's gone AWOL, don't worry. It may have dissolved or been pushed out without your knowledge. Douche with plain water and drink a quart of water to let peristalsis coax it out. If it's the whole gauze and string creation that's stuck inside, wait a day to see if it comes out.

In all the years since women have been self-treating this way and telling me about it, I have never heard of a case in which garlic actually festered deep inside. But I have heard a few doctors say that this happens. So if, after using a garlic suppository, you develop sudden severe pains, a high fever, malaise, or other signs of an acute infection, or if you can't stop worrying about it, see your health care provider.

In self-treating for intestinal yeast, some women report good results from similar use of rectal suppositories of garlic overnight for two weeks. That *cannot* get stuck or cause problems, even if constipation is a concern, due to the pH and environment of the colon. Garlic can only help our digestive immune-system cells there, with sulfur-rich compounds to kill off fungi and "bad" bacteria.

External Herbal Formula II

Commiphora mol-mol (myrrh resin powder)   1 ounce
Calendula officinalis (calendula flowers)   1 ounce

Powder the lightweight calendula flowers in a clean coffee grinder. Stir together with myrrh powder. Make a compound tincture with alcohol of at least 100 proof (50% alcohol); see Chapter 2: Herbal Preparation. Dilute one tablespoon per 8-ounce container of filtered, "clean" water. Tap water has bacteria and microbes in it, so boil it for at least fifteen minutes, then allow it to cool. Use this douche (diluted tincture) every three to four days for three weeks.

Please don't douche more than four times a week—preferably no more than twice in one week. Natural defenses shouldn't be rinsed away more than necessary. A more lasting health improvement can be made by taking herbs internally, making good food choices, and changing immune-system function by reducing stress.

There are other herbal treatments besides douching that can be used as needed for symptom relief. It is all right to treat symptoms every day, depending on severity, if we also treat the underlying cause.

If treatment continues longer than three weeks, alternate the above formula every other week with the following:

External Herbal Formula III

Juglans nigra (black walnut hulls)   3 teaspoons
Melaleuca alternifolia (ti tree essential oil)   6–10 drops
water   9 ounces

Make an 8-ounce cup of tea by simmering 3 teaspoons of black walnut hulls in just over 1 cup of boiling water (see Chapter 2: Herbal Preparation). Allow tea to cool to a comfortable temperature; while it is still warm, stir in 6–10 drops of ti tree oil. Oil and water don't mix well, so if droplets of oil can be seen on the surface of the tea, whisk the mixture together. Use this to rinse the labia one to two times a day, making sure to wash those tender folds. Repeat the process every day as needed.

Depending on the severity of itching and related symptoms, or if your time schedule just can't handle using herbs internally and externally several days in a row, there is a quick symptom treatment. However, both the severity of symptoms and the packed schedule too many days in a row may be signs that you need to slow your life down. For the "desperate woman," wash your hands and under your finger-nails *very well* before taking two or three drops of marjoram or ti tree essential oil on your fingertips. Insert your fingertips into the first inch of the vaginal canal and swab lightly around. Wash your hands again. The essential oil may smart on inflamed lesions of yeast, but after a half-minute of sharp in-breaths and jumping up and down, women report that this buys hours of symptomatic relief from severe itching and discomfort. The essential oils are killing off yeast and fungal growth without harming the delicate epithelial membranes of your vagina, so the infection clears up rapidly. This is not sufficient by itself to get to the root of the infection, however.

Nutrition

Several books on candida and diet are available, but it can be problematic to live with the advice. The recommendations of a whole-food diet low in sugars is good. But everyone is different, and there are those who don't respond as well as others to a strict eating plan. It isn't healing to develop extreme beliefs regarding what is to be let in and what is excluded. Eating next to nothing because of fear creates sick bodies. Candida diets may be better with some cleansing and vitamin-rich immune system–boosting foods, *including* fruit.

A reasonable rule to follow when starting the healing process is to give the body a chance to normalize an imbalance of blood sugar. Avoid all processed sugars, in-cluding honey, natural sweeteners, and tropical fruit (citrus, bananas, all fruit juices). The focus needs to remain on a balance between cleansing and detoxifica-tion on one hand, and rebuilding and nourishing what is *not* sick. I am not con-vinced that organic apple cider vinegar, all fruit, every form of yeast, and all mushrooms are "wrong" foods, unless there is a food allergy. When even small amounts of nourishing whole foods give intestinal gas, bloating or vaginal flare-ups of candida symptoms, it may be that the digestive system is low in the strong stom-ach acid required for disinfecting and breaking down food. This is why many anti-candida herbs stimulate good digestive function. Bloating might also indicate that one's digestive system has not seen a particular food in so long that it needs time to create the necessary enzymes for thorough metabolism. More than anything else, our immune system and digestive system want gradual dietary changes and rou-tine. You may be adventurous, but your stomach is happiest with routine: similar whole foods in small amounts at the same time each day, in a relaxed schedule re-peated over many days. Candida doesn't go away by eating "health food" take-out packaged foods, washed down with natural sodas, while sitting at a desk or driving a car.

Garlic is an excellent antifungal. Raw, steamed, or cooked, you should eat one to three cloves each day if you have candida, unless you cannot tolerate it because of digestive upsets or a breast-feeding baby with colic. Odorless products are available but are less effective against infections.

Prepare seaweeds (2 ounces dry: dulse, kelp, hijiki, kombu, sea fronds) twice a week or more.

Mix equal parts of dried, sifted *Urtica dioica* (nettle leaf) with ground seaweeds or other herbs and spices, to taste. Use 2 ounces per week as seasoning in soups, in salads, and over cooked grains. If fresh spring shoots are available in your area, steam 3–6 ounces three times a week during the early growing season. Eating nettles is highly nutritious, but after late spring, shoots and young leaves develop tiny hairs that are irritating to the mouth and throat. If you miss the shoots in early spring, make tea from dried leaves.

Whole grains are helpful because they have B-vitamins and fiber for colon cleansing. But don't overeat complex carbohydrates—and avoid refined flour products—unless you are burning the fuel with high levels of activity.

Eat temperate-zone raw fruits (apples, pears, plums, peaches) in moderation and in season. Two a day, eaten slowly and chewed thoroughly, give you the fiber needed to clear candida and other problem microbes from your intestines.

Supplements

Raw acidophilus: With high counts of live, "good" bacteria, this replaces healthy flora lost due to use of antibiotics or other immunosuppression. It is available at health food stores in liquid or capsule form. Take as directed on labels.

Caprylic acid: a natural supplement that is specific to fighting candida. Because this comes in different strengths, follow recommended doses on labels.

Grapefruit seed extract: follow recommended doses or labels.

Other Points

Plain (unflavored) live-culture yogurt has been used successfully for many years as a vaginal antifungal. If the yogurt comes with fruit in the bottom and preservatives, or sugar and gelatin, it isn't fit to put in your mouth *or* your vagina. Live yogurt culture has bacteria that are "friendly" to our vaginal bacteria yet kill off the opportunistic yeast. Cool yogurt is soothing on puffy, painful vaginal tissues.

However, if one teaspoon of yogurt inserted once or twice a day for three days has not resolved the problem, the thready arms of the fungus may be reaching deeper into the tissues, requiring more penetrating antimicrobial herbs with a more specific effect on recurrent or chronic fungi and yeast infections.

20
Herpes

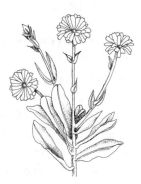

Definition

Herpes genitalis, also known as Herpes simplex virus II (HSV), is a sexually transmitted disease. Herpes simplex virus I may also cause the lesions associated with this viral infection. It is so common now as to be virtually epidemic. Herpes is a chronic viral infection of the nerve tissues that may flare up during periods of high stress or lowered immunity. It may manifest on the skin or genitalia as a painful open sore. Herpes can be handled herbally, but neither herbs nor prescription antiviral drugs can promise to remove the virus, as far as we know. Yet there is hope for a healthy life. People have gone ten years or longer without one outbreak, even under stress; but this is not proof that the virus is gone. Treatment only reduces the viral population to a great degree.

Symptoms and Signs

Within three to seven days after exposure, painless bumps filled with fluid appear somewhere on the genitalia of either gender. Sores can also appear around the anal region or on the mouth. When these bumps erupt, they become shallow, painful, red ulcers. The center oozes fluid, and local lymph nodes usually become enlarged and tender because the immune system is trying to contain the spread of the infection.

There may also be general signs of infection, such as fever, tiredness, painful urination, or a white vaginal discharge. Some people also suffer muscle aches and pains.

Repeat occurrences often announce their arrival with a tingling sensation where old lesions have been. There can be several stages of lesions beginning, closing, or fading all at once. Any lesion on the surface of the body means that a person is potentially contagious. Avoiding sex during these periods is crucial, as is treatment for partners.

Common discomforts include the itchy lesions on genital and surrounding tissue, as well as the notorious state of tension that closely precedes or follows an outbreak. In women, the symptoms often begin with a tingling sensation where the sore will be, unless it can be stopped in its tracks. The virus commonly manifests in the vulva, especially the labia majora. The virus isn't just in the tissue; it stays dormant in the nerves, allowing the virus to manifest on the surface of the reproductive tissues as a tingling patch or lesion under stressful conditions. Less commonly, it may show up elsewhere in the reproductive tract or pubic area. Lymph nodes in the groin may swell and feel tender or painful.

Cause

Herpes is usually transmitted sexually, but occasionally it can be passed from contagious lesions through towels, bathtubs, and toilet seats. If a pregnant woman has a contagious herpes lesion, the virus can be passed to the baby during vaginal delivery.

Conventional Medical Care

The orthodox view is that the viral infection lasts for life. The flare-ups are inflammatory but self-limiting. However, if a woman's age is advanced or her immunity is weakened, the genital lesions may lead to painful local or systemic disease.

Without treatment, lesions located elsewhere than the genitals can lead to serious complications. Inflammation from herpes can lead to blindness or even death, but this is rare.

The standard antiviral is Acyclovir, also called Zovirax, though others are used. Ointment for external use is combined with pills. Severe herpes in people who have compromised immune systems may be treated with intravenous Acyclovir or other antiviral drugs.

Because herpes can occur on the cervix, all women with risk of exposure or a previous diagnosis of herpes are encouraged to have a Pap smear twice a year. Herpes may disguise gonorrhea or even predispose women to cervical cancer, which is a chronic degenerative disease with overlapping risk factors for chronic venereal infections.

Pain-relieving sprays or ointments such as Xylocaine are often given for symptom relief, along with recommendations to switch from soap to oatmeal products such as Aveeno bars or soaks.

Herbal Treatment

The holistic objective is not to suppress or eradicate the virus, but to decrease outbreaks and their triggers, including stress. Herbs are used to restore the normal function of nerve tissue. Women can introduce specific antiviral herbs while increasing their nonspecific resistance to viral expression. The goal is to stop having contagious and painful outbreaks, even though the virus is there. While several herbs used for treating herpes are known to be antiviral, these herbs have other actions to lessen painful outbreaks of herpes lesions. For example, *Hypericum perforatum* (St. Johnswort) is also anti-inflammatory and is a nervine tonic to the nervous system.

Herpes II is often associated with HPV (Human Papilloma Virus), with or without genital warts or dysplasia (abnormal cervical cell growth). As with the example of St. Johnswort, many of the herbs in the following formula help the person with herpes, rather than just fighting the herpes or HPV.

Herbal Formula I

Hypericum perforatum (St. Johnswort herb)	4 ounces
Calendula officinalis (calendula flower)	2 ounces
Turnera diffusa (damiana herb)	1 ounce
Echinacea spp. (echinacea root)	2 ounces
Baptisia tinctoria (wild indigo root)	1 ounce
Eleutherococcus senticosus (Siberian ginseng root)	1 ounce
Anemone pulsatilla (pasque flower; flower, herb)	3 ounces

Steep 1 ounce of this mixture in 2 pints of boiling water for 20 minutes. Strain, and drink one large glass three times a day, for a minimum of ten days. Alternatively, combine these as extracts, and take 1 teaspoon four times a day for five days a week. Continue for one to three months as needed; consultation with an herbalist is advised.

If anxiety and episodes of stress worsen outbreaks, add:

Scutellaria lateriflora (skullcap herb)	1 ounce
Humulus lupulus (hops flower)	½ ounce

Increase Siberian ginseng to 3 ounces in cases of severe chronic stress that cannot be changed.

If the hormonal imbalance of menses worsens herpes outbreaks, add:

Vitex agnus-castus (chasteberry seed)	2 ounces
Smilax ornata (sarsaparilla root)	1 ounce

The Siberian ginseng in Herbal Formula I is an *adaptogen*; it increases nonspecific resistance, allowing people to manage stress more easily. Calendula is both antiviral and a lymphatic remedy, promoting lymph flow and function.

Echinacea is generally antimicrobial (specifically antiviral here), and it increases the number of leukocytes (white blood cells) and their activity. Research suggests that echinacea works, in part, by protecting the matrix of connective tissue (made of hyaluronic acid) against infection. Echinacea does this by neutralizing the enzyme *hyaluronidase* produced by invading microbes. This prevents the microbe from penetrating the cell contents. While this does not explain its antiviral effects against herpes, it shows that antiviral herbs are more than antiviral compounds.

Turnera diffusa (damiana) is a relaxing nervine and tonic with an affinity for nervous system problems that affect the reproductive system. (This aromatic Mexican herb was called *Turnera aphrodisiaca* before botanists got worried that people would get the wrong idea and toned down the Latin name.) Damiana works by increasing blood flow, blood oxygenation, and energy in the affected area while it relaxes the whole person. In Herbal Formula I, it is given in too small an amount to cause sexual arousal. It does increase one's sense of well-being, which is central to vibrant immunity.

Two other valuable nervines in Herbal Formula I are *Anemone pulsatilla* (pasque flower herb) and *Avena sativa* (oat straw). *Smilax* is an alterative (detoxifying herb) with anti-inflammatory sterols. The antivirals against herpes work most effectively in combination with such nonspecific herbal remedies.

Symptoms such as painful lesions should respond in one to two days even though it takes longer for them to heal completely. Fatigue and swollen lymph nodes may take three to seven days to respond. It will take one to three months of consistent use of herbs internally, along with nutritional and other changes, to reduce outbreaks. If these herbal treatments have little or no effect, get a clear diagnosis and treatment from a qualified practitioner.

During pregnancy, the focus of Herbal Formula II is on prevention with immune-system support rather than on strong antivirals. Also see "Herpes" in Chapter 15: Pregnancy.

Herbal Formula II for Pregnancy

Rubus idaeus (raspberry leaf)	3 ounces
Avena sativa (oat straw herb)	2 ounces

Echinacea spp. (echinacea root)	4 ounces
Urtica dioica (nettle leaf)	2 ounces
Anemone pulsatilla (pasque flower; flower, herb)	2 ounces
Melissa officinalis (lemon balm herb)	4 ounces
Scutellaria lateriflora (skullcap herb)	1 ounce

Steep 1 ounce of this mixture in 2 pints of boiling water for 20 minutes; strain tea. Drink one 12- to 16-ounce glass a day for a minimum of two weeks. For longer-term use if needed, lower the amount of echinacea to 2 ounces. Continue for one to three months as needed; consultation with your health care provider and an herbalist is advised. Note: Since pregnant women are sensitive to flavor, lemon balm is optional; it is considered antiviral, it settles digestive upsets, and it tastes good to most pregnant women.

External Herbal Therapies

Keep the area dry except when applying antiviral ointment or herbal preparations for disinfecting and drying bumps or lesions. These can be used to soothe the itching or irritation of the skin before a lesion appears, but in all cases be scrupulous about washing your hands to prevent the spread of infection.

Choose one of the following for symptom relief of lesions (apply to lesions with a sterile swab or Q-tip):

- lysine cream, available in most natural food stores
- St. Johnswort tincture
- licorice tincture
- calendula tincture
- lavender essential oil

The alcohol in the tinctures will sting initially, but this is the best way to dry open lesions rapidly. Apply one to five times per day, as needed. The lavender essential oil alternative has two benefits: less burning and an additional aromatherapy effect of lifting the spirits. The three tinctures can be combined in equal parts, applied topically every few hours for effective, rapid results.

Nutrition

Foods that worsen herpes symptoms are high in the amino acid arginine, which has been shown to be used by the herpes virus to replicate. Another amino acid, lysine, helps prevent herpes outbreaks by blocking the body's use of arginine. Four ounces of fresh fish (grilled, steamed, baked—not raw) is almost equal to two 500-milligram lysine tablets. Halibut and lean white fish may have higher lysine content than other varieties of fish. The following lists can help you increase your intake of lysine-rich foods, and decrease your intake of arginine (refer to a nutrition almanac for more complete lists).

Food Sources of Lysine

4 ounces	fresh fish	930 milligrams
	canned fish	810
	chicken	740
	goat's milk	520
½ cup	cooked mung beans	410
	cooked beans, various	270

The following foods contain both lysine and arginine, but they have more harmful arginine than protective lysine, causing a "lysine deficiency." For example, you can more than compensate for the arginine in ½ cup of brown rice (approximately equal to -190 milligrams lysine deficiency) with ½ cup of cooked lentils (270 milligrams lysine).

Food Sources of Arginine

		Producing a Lysine Deficiency of:
½ cup	hazel nuts	-2,250 milligrams
	brazil nuts	-2,110
	peanuts	-2,060
	walnuts	-810
	almonds	-710
	cocoa powder	-650
2 tablespoons	peanut butter	-510
½ cup	sesame seeds	-450
	brown rice	-190
4 slices	whole wheat bread	-160
½ cup	cooked oatmeal	-130
	raisins	-130
	sunflower seeds	-130

Note: Moderate daily use (1–3 teaspoons) of sesame seeds, sunflower seeds, or flax seed oil can be beneficial, though these contain some arginine. The essential fatty acids have immune-system and cellular repair functions, so they are worth eating even though they contain some arginine.

Herpes appears to be antagonized by garlic. Eat lots of it (one to four cloves a day), raw or steamed in the diet, to taste. If garlic causes gas or other gastric distress, try supplements (following).

Avoid refined sugars and caffeine, and limit your intake of citrus to one piece of fresh fruit daily.

Supplements

During outbreaks, some women find it helpful to take lysine capsules (500 milligrams, 4–6 daily). In severe cases, a maintenance dose is one capsule three times a day for one to three months, followed by one capsule once a day for another one to three months.

Daily recommendations include:

vitamin A: 25,000 IU

beta-Carotene: 2,500 milligrams

vitamin C: 500 milligrams–10 grams (or to bowel tolerance; when more vitamin C is taken than one needs, it may soften the stool, and may even lead to temporary diarrhea)

kelp tablets: 6 with food if seaweed is not available

deodorized garlic tablets or perles: 6 with food (if not eaten in the diet)

Other Points

Swim in the ocean or add Epsom salt to your bath; salt water dries sores. Epsom salt is available in drug stores.

Sitz baths (frequent and hot) improve circulation to the area. Replace soap with ¼ cup of plain rolled oatmeal flakes as a soothing skin scrub. Place dry oats in a muslin bag or cotton sock (old pantyhose tied off at one end will work); use in hot bath water like a sponge to slough off dead skin cells while milky oats moisturize dry or inflamed skin. Oatmeal baths also reduce itching.

Exercise relieves tension and brings herbs to problem areas through improved circulation. Whether dancing alone in your room, strolling in fresh air, or joining in group sports, choose movement for fun as well as "health benefits." A break in routine should feel like an adventure, if not a vacation!

Keep the genital area dry during the day; wear cotton underwear. Avoid tight-fitting clothes.

21

Trichomonas

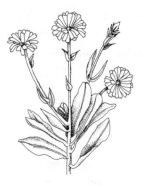

Definition

Trichomoniasis also commonly known as trichomonas, is one of the common types of vaginitis, an inflammation of the vaginal linings. It is usually a sexually transmitted disease (STD). *Trichomonas vaginalis* is the parasitic organism responsible—not to be confused with *trichinosis,* the infestation of worms that can result from eating uncooked pork.

Symptoms and Signs

This protozoan (a one-celled microorganism) causes more intense symptoms of vaginal itching, irritation, and discharge than bacteria, candida, or even viruses. The thin vaginal discharge is yellow to green. It may have small bubbles of air, giving a frothy appearance, and the discharge burns on the raw vaginal lining. The infection makes sex painful. It has a characteristic bad smell, unlike the yeasty smell of candida or the fishy-smelling, cream-to-gray discharge of *Gardnerella* or BV, an infection caused by a specific bacterium.

Trichomoniasis also causes painful urination when urine passes inflamed vaginal tissues. There may also be frequent urination and spasm upon urination.

General signs of infection may be present, such as a fever, chills, nausea, fatigue, or irritability. Trichomoniasis can mimic a bladder infection (cystitis). The organism can live in the tissue of the vagina or the urethra, or hidden away inside Bartholin's glands located on either side of the vagina, deep in the tissue. When trichomoniasis occurs as a chronic infection, symptoms are less obvious but may flare up suddenly, especially getting worse during menstrual periods. The infection can also mask gonorrhea, so an infection that does not clear up with herbal treatment must be referred to a licensed practitioner.

Cause

Trichomoniasis is caused by a microorganism called a *trichomonad*. The trichomonad is a one-celled simple life form with four tails. The tails, called *flagellae* (singular: *flagella*), move the protozoa around. The group of organisms these trichomonads belong to are called *flagellates.*

Contact with this flagellate is usually through sexual intercourse with an infected partner. Men may carry the protozoa without symptoms. Reinfection of partners is common.

Conventional Medical Care

The conventional treatment is with one or repeated courses of Flagyl (metronidazole), which is also used to treat vaginitis caused by *Gardnerella*. Flagyl, like some of the strong herbs used to treat protozoal infection, is not safe to use during pregnancy or breast-feeding. No other conventional medicine is used during pregnancy, at least until after the second trimester, although vaginal tablets of another drug, Clotrimazole, may be prescribed.

Flagyl's drawbacks include side effects such as a metal taste in the mouth, coated tongue, headaches, nausea, vomiting, or abdominal cramps. Some people are allergic to it. In rare cases, it can cause neurological problems, such as numbness, tingling in the fingers and toes, or convulsions. Drug reactions such as allergic rash are not uncommon.

Taking Flagyl is commonly perceived, by women who take it and some health care workers who prescribe it, to fail as often as it works. It has been suggested by conventional medical personnel that it may give a temporary false negative reading. If Flagyl *does* kill the protozoa, it leaves women with yeast infections afterward or in the near future because it suppresses the woman's immune system. If it is used, follow with acidophilus or live yogurt.

All sexual partners must be treated during a period of abstinence to prevent reinfection and spread. Because Flagyl is not uniformly effective at killing off the protozoa, it is recommended that you be tested after treatment to be sure the infection has been resolved.

For irritation, vaginal ointments with corticosteroids may be prescribed.

Herbal Treatment

This difficult creature is resistant to treatment. It takes a while to clear with herbs. Neither conventional nor herbal antimicrobial therapies for trichomoniasis are recommended during pregnancy. During pregnancy, herbs can limit damage from infections until after delivery, when stronger antiprotozoal compounds (conventional or herbal) may be used to get beyond symptoms to the cause.

The holistic objective in treating trichomoniasis is to eliminate protozoan microorganisms while optimizing natural immune-system defenses against recurrence. Prevention of recurrence includes eliminating risk factors, primarily unsafe sex. Condoms are required until both or all partners test negative. Women partners may be tested to see if they require treatment.

The herbal treatment usually requires a consistent two months before a retest is considered reliable, and it is preferable to err on the side of caution. Repeat the test twice: two weeks after all symptoms are gone and once again three weeks later.

One of the best herbal antiprotozoals for treating trichomoniasis is *Picrasma excelsa* (quassia bark, pronounced "KWA-see-ya" or "KWAH-shah"). Other herbs used to treat the person with this stubborn infection may not depend on antiprotozoal effects alone. They include *Commiphora spp.* (myrrh resin) and *Berberis vulgaris* (barberry root bark, not "bearberry," a leaf used to treat urinary tract infections). Hepatic herbs help if the liver is already compromised from taking Flagyl. This drug is so frequently repeated in normal practice before doctors and patients give up on it that liver herbs such as barberry may be needed for effective healing. Others needed may include tonics for long-term immune-system benefits; two examples are *Ganoderma spp.* (reishi mushrooms) and *Astragalus membranaceus* (huang chi root), depending on individual need.

Herbal Formula I

Picrasma excelsa (quassia root)	4 ounces
Berberis vulgaris (barberry root bark)	3 ounces
Echinacea spp. (purple coneflower root, seed)	2 ounces
Baptisia indigo (wild indigo root)	1 ounce
Passiflora incarnata (passionflower herb)	3 ounces
Artemisia annua (sweet Annie herb)	1 ounce

The herbs strong enough to kill protozoal microorganisms are herbs that nature designed to taste particularly vile. If you cannot afford to buy tincture, you should make this formula as a compound tincture at home (please see Chapter 2: Herbal Preparation; herbs and alcohol must sit for two weeks before tincture is ready). Meanwhile, this formula tastes so bad as a tea that capsules are the only other option for humane oral administration. The mixture can be ground in a coffee grinder at home and capped (see Chapter 2: Herbal Preparation). The dose for capsules is two #00 capsules taken with water four times a day; continue for six weeks.

Note: Some herbs in this formula are not safe for use during pregnancy. Please see Chapter 15 for safe antimicrobials.

These strong herbs are not as bad as repeated courses of immune-system-suppressing drugs. Skip herbs one day per week if you are taking this formula for three months.

If your immunity is poor, if you repeat treatment twice in one year, or if treatment continues longer than three months, add the following herbs:

Silybum marianum (also called *Carduus marianum*) (milk thistle seed)	3 ounces
Ganoderma lucidum (reishi mushroom)	3 ounces

Alternatively, either of these two herbs can be taken as separate extracts according to directions on labels.

Formula I may be taken along with prescription drugs (for trichomoniasis or other reasons). If there is cramping or other side effects from either conventional drugs or herbs, a separate herbal tea (Formula II) that is both soothing to the digestion and delicious can be taken as often as needed.

Herbal Formula II

Althaea officinalis (marshmallow root)	1 ounce
Hibiscus spp. (hibiscus flowers)	2 ounces
Taraxacum officinale (dandelion root, roasted)	2 ounces

Use standard preparation and dose, as needed for digestive disturbances. If you prefer, substitute your favorite herb flavors such as fennel, peppermint, or lemon balm.

External Herbal Therapies

Herbal Formula for Douche and Wash

Picrasma excelsa (quassia root bark)	4 ounces
Larrea mexicana (chaparral herb)	4 ounces

For two partners, simmer 4 ounces of this mixture in one gallon of water for thirty minutes on low heat. Strain herbs out and return tea to a clean pan and simmer, partially covered, on low heat. Evaporate down to one-third gallon. Store in refrigerator. Warm ½ cup at a time for douching or washing external genitalia completely every day.

This is a good opportunity for a male partner to enjoy a penis soak, using ½ cup of the external herbal preparation above. The masculine equivalent of a douche, this involves submerging one's penis in the herbal liquid, in a jar or other comfortably sized container, for fifteen minutes. Yes, it is ridiculous, but now men can share some of the laughs and the hassle of natural self-help for STDs.

Nutrition

What one eats is not paramount in the herbal treatment of this persistent infection because it is not linked to poor diet. However, stress on the liver from the conventional drugs may be offset with low-protein, high-quality whole foods. Following a good whole-food plan is always beneficial when killing off one type of infecting organism and building up one's health and immunity.

Other Points

Avoid sex until partners are clear of trichomoniasis and any additional STDs according to diagnostic tests. If herbal treatment or conventional medical care does not clear this infection, do not give up. See a licensed practitioner.

22

Chlamydia

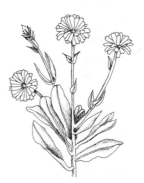

Definition

The most common STD in North America, chlamydia is caused by a one-celled parasite with a rigid cell wall. This makes it harder to clear up with vaginal application of herbs. *Chlamydia trachomatis* is one of the common causes of urethritis in men and cervicitis in women. It often goes undiagnosed. This partly explains why it is the leading cause of more serious pelvic disease in women, particularly acute salpingitis (infected fallopian tubes).

Symptoms and Signs

Symptoms appear long after contact, so transmission happens easily. Chlamydia is also difficult to diagnose for the simple reason that it takes different forms in different individuals. There may be no symptoms, or symptoms might look like any number of other conditions.

A painless bump often goes unnoticed, though it may be followed in one to four weeks by swollen lymph glands, headache, joint and muscle pain, chills, and weight loss. There may be vaginal discharge that feels like mucus and has a bad odor. A woman may complain of pain with sexual intercourse, or even a little spotting of blood after sex. An inflamed cervix may also lead to spotting between menstrual periods; a licensed practitioner may look for signs of redness on the cervix. Moving the cervix or touching its surface may cause pain (this doesn't normally hurt).

Systemic signs include a slight fever, urinary frequency or painful urination, and lower abdominal pain. One's sexual partner may have had urethritis in the past. An inflamed urethra with a burning sensation in men or women is most commonly due to chlamydia, though urethritis may be caused by gonorrhea or other organisms.

Untreated, chlamydia can lead to complications such as acute infections of the reproductive system, pelvic inflammatory disease, and sterility. In women, the obstruction of lymph nodes may cause swelling or even discharge. Secondary or repeated infections with scarring can cause abscesses or *fistulas* (in which infective material erupts from one body compartment to another, or out on the skin).

In pregnancy, chlamydia can cause premature or difficult delivery, or infection of the child during passage through the birth canal. Especially in less industrialized nations than the United States, chlamydia causes blindness in babies and even death.

Men infected with chlamydia may have tender, enlarged inguinal lymph nodes (in the groin). Untreated, this will worsen. Most herbalists would not be called upon to treat these serious consequences of late-stage chlamydia infection. This is fortunate, because most don't have the necessary tools to help at this stage.

A swab from the site of infection is cultured from a patient with salpingitis (inflamed fallopian tubes), cervicitis (inflamed cervix), urethritis (inflamed urethra), or other genitourinary inflammation. Culture of other body fluids confirms the diagnosis.

Cause

Chlamydia can be spread by exposure to the organism in the genitalia or anal region. It can also be passed orally.

Conventional Medical Care

In conventional drug treatment, antibiotics such as Doxycycline or Erythromycin are given for one to two weeks, depending on the circumstances and whether this is a new or repeat infection, or whether a woman with chlamydia is pregnant. Secondary infections with viruses, bacteria, and yeasts may result from antibiotic treatment and require additional holistic care for prevention or a complete return to health. Once chlamydia is diagnosed, tests for other STDs are given.

Herbal Treatment

Herbs used to treat women who have chlamydia are parasiticides with other immune system–supportive properties. These may be combined for the individual using any one or more of the following nonspecific remedies: the antiviral anti-inflammatory *Calendula*, antibacterial *Commiphora* (myrrh), antimicrobial *Berberis* species, demulcents such as *Plantago lanceolata*, external vulneraries such as *Symphytum,* reproductive astringent tonics and hormonal normalizing agents *Rubus idaeus* and *Caulophyllum*, and penetrating antiseptics such as essential oil of *Melaleuca spp.* (ti tree) and the warming *Tropaeolum majus* (nasturtium).

Note that many of these herbs are not safe for use during pregnancy. Those strong enough to kill off parasites in the following herbal formula are absolutely contraindicated during pregnancy. If two safe antimicrobials in pregnancy, echinacea and garlic, don't work in standard doses (as prescribed in Chapter16: Pregnancy), Erythromycin would be safer than the following formula during pregnancy. At other times, the antibiotics and following herbs will not counteract each other, so both may be taken at the same time. The goal is to get a clear culture from each sexual partner after treatment.

Herbal Formula

Berberis vulgaris (barberry root bark)	6 ounces

Because this is a two-step process, store the barberry separately from the next three herbs:

Inula helenium (elecampane root)	4 ounces
Thymus vulgaris (thyme herb)	1 ounce
Tanacetum vulgare (tansy flower, leaf)	1 ounce

Simmer ½ ounce of barberry in 3 cups of water, covered, for fifteen minutes. Turn off heat, add ½ ounce of the mixture of the three remaining herbs. Cover and let steep for another ten minutes. Strain the tea. It will taste quite bitter. For each dose, dilute ¾ cup with ¾ cup black cherry juice or water to taste. Drink two to three doses a day, depending on how much tea (1½–2¼ cups or so) is strained from the original three cups of water (¾ cup or so is left in the wet herbs). Repeat for ten to fourteen days whether symptoms are present or not.

To prevent reinfection it is necessary to treat all partners and stress the importance of avoiding sexual contact until the course of treatment is complete. If partners are men, don't count on condoms alone to prevent transmission.

If there are any feelings of abdominal pain or tender lymph nodes in the groin after treatment, see a health care provider.

External Herbal Therapies

Though this book frequently lists an herbal douche for reproductive infections, these are not advisable for anything but short-term symptom relief while the cause of vaginal imbalance is being addressed through changes in nutrition and internal herbal support.

We cannot rely on douching except to temporarily relieve symptoms and improve the quality of life. Douching rinses away helpful vaginal lubrication, such as the enzyme-rich mucus that traps potential problem germs. Though antimicrobial herbs used vaginally may help a women to get a jump-start on reducing inappropriate microorganisms, douching removes healthy flora, which normally create the acidic secretions that prevent colonization of common opportunistic yeasts. Repeated application of water in douching is eventually drying, making the irritated vaginal wall more susceptible to infections. Having said that, temporary use of the following external formula helps clear the chlamydia:

Herbal Formula for Douche

Calendula officinalis (calendula flower)	1 ounce
Berberis aquifolium (Oregon grape root)	2 ounces
ti tree essential oil	1 teaspoon

Steep 1 ounce of a mixture of the first two herbs only, in one pint of boiling water, covered, for 45 minutes or until cooled to a comfortable temperature for vaginal use. Strain tea. Add 1 teaspoon of essential oil (approximately 5–7 drops of essential oil per ounce of tea). Mix well and douche; hold in for five minutes twice a day. Repeat twice a week for three weeks. It is not necessary to rinse.

PART SIX

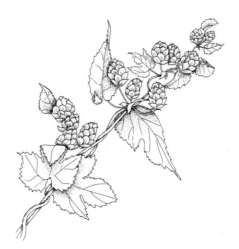

The Change of Life

23

Menopause

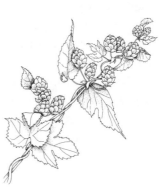

Definition

Menopause occurs when our ovaries have finished releasing eggs. This simple biological change in normal function has been made complex by Western society's perception that change and age are bad. The female human body has been designed for millennia to slow estrogen production at this time. Menopause is not a disease requiring treatment; the change of life is a natural rite of transformation. "The Change" is another name for menopause, symbolic of the truth that "all is change" in life.

Menopause is a *pause,* or end, to our *menses.* The average length of time during which menopause takes place is just over a year. When we no longer menstruate, we are said to hold that rhythm inside us instead of giving it away every month. You are officially "done" with menstruation when one to two years without bleeding or pregnancy have passed. Menopause seems a better term than the medical term, *climacteric,* which implies that since our reproductive years have reached a climax, we can only expect to go downhill from there. At this age, we are free to travel, finally getting those important letters written, and accomplish profound transformation, social activism, or contemplation.

All theories about what menopause should be like are irrelevant. The essential key for women is to examine, reassess, and contemplate their relationship with others and their world. All that any woman's body asks of her is that she pay attention. Her spirit asks that she open to new resources of support, inspiration, and purpose.

The occurrence of menopause is unique to human females; no other animal goes through it. It may be that, in past eras, large numbers of women didn't live long enough to spend much time living through and past menopause. There have never been so many women of this age, surviving for so long in a world running wild with instant communication and self-analysis. Women in menopause are now living long enough, and in great enough numbers, to learn new roles of power that are nonreproductive. This is changing our understanding of what "normal" menopause means.

Natural menopause can occur from thirty-six to sixty years of age, with the average age being about fifty-one years at the time of onset. In other cultures, where girls bear children at a young age, thirty-six is not considered an unhealthy age for menopause, though it is considered premature in the West, especially if it is triggered by some form of ill health.

Symptoms and Signs

Out of the thirty to forty million women going through the Change at this time in the United States, many have no negative signs or symptoms. Yet we mainly hear horror stories about menopausal women—who are, in fact, at the extreme ends of the range of normal "problems." There is said to be "loss of control" over body temperature and "abnormal" emotional swings. In fact, there is no loss of control, but there is a change in the body's thermostat for physical and emotional self-control. With menopausal symptoms comes an awareness of the mortality of one's physical body. This can be liberating or frightening, depending on a woman's beliefs. As many as eighty percent of women who have noticeable signs and symptoms experience a fairly normal menopause; ten percent have no signs at all, and ten percent have severe health breakdown related to the Change.

Some symptoms of menopause are positive: On their own, menstrual migraines and estrogen-dependent growths, including fibroids, lessen or even disappear because the estrogen level decreases.

Another popular belief that is *not* helpful to women is that healthy women have no symptoms of menopause. This misconception seems to be that anything as natural as menopause should be a snap. I'm sure we're all familiar with this illusory ideal: the superwoman who does everything right, is in perfect health because she eats all her vegetables, enjoys emotional equilibrium because she creates art instead of repressing her feelings, and sails through menopause without a rough patch. While it is true that vegetables help, and many women have a lovely menopause without trauma or medication, it is important that real women are given help. Their needs are not to be trivialized.

Holistic treatment of menopausal women looks at seven interconnected symptoms and the body systems they involve:

1. hot flashes (cardiovascular system—CVS)

2. osteoporosis (musculoskeletal system)

3. vaginal dryness or atrophy, which may lead to increased incidence of cystitis (reproductive and urinary systems)

4. irregular cycle, heavy bleeding, and spotting (reproductive system)

5. increased cardiovascular system risk simultaneous with low estrogen level (reproductive and cardiovascular systems)

6. dysmenorrhea, often with characteristic "dragging" sensations (nervous and reproductive systems)

7. aches and pains, arthritic changes with age, changing pain threshold, and related depression (nervous system and musculoskeletal system)

These are the seven main areas of overlapping concerns, although the digestive system and other body systems may also be affected during menopause, especially blood sugar level and thyroid function (endocrine system).

Hot Flashes

For many women, hot flashes are the most debilitating symptom of menopause, though both the symptom and the cause respond well to natural care. Think of hot flashes as power surges. The blood vessel changes are a mirror of your innermost physical being. This is your feminine spirit in the chemical form of a hormone. It wants your undivided attention to remind you to rest, eat something else, take a walk, change your mind.

The hot flash begins in the brain. The hypothalamus controls body temperature and estrogen levels. When the estrogen level starts to drop in an uneven stop-and-start sort of way, the hypothalamus sends a chemical messenger (gonadotropin releasing hormone, or GnRH) to the pituitary gland (located behind the "third eye" between the eyes, deep in the brain). The front half of the pituitary gland sends follicle stimulating hormone (FSH) to the ovaries, requesting that they please come up with some more estrogen. The ovaries may or may not comply, depending on whether there are any viable egg follicles left in the ovaries to stimulate. When an egg follicle in the ovary develops, it makes estrogen levels in the bloodstream rise, satisfying the hypothalamus and the pituitary. But eventually, as we approach menopause, a woman's eggs are all used up and the ovary cannot comply with orders from upstairs.

This mirrors times in a woman's outer life, when she is ordered to do a job "as usual" but doesn't have the required tools and materials. It's not a failure; it's time for new instructions from headquarters.

Frustrated, the body's hormonal system responds to continuing low levels of estrogen by trying to "storm" the hypothalamus with adrenaline to get it moving. In turn, this will goose the ovaries into action. This tempest in a teapot affects the hypothalamus's temperature-control center. Now the body's thermostat control is reset for a lower temperature, like turning down the control on central heating. Women may actually feel a little chill.

The heart responds to adrenaline's effect on the hypothalamus; the heart rate speeds up a little or a lot, depending on the woman or the strength of the hot flash.

Now the skin gets involved. All the blood vessels from the heart to the skin have a sophisticated way of bringing the body temperature down to the new level set by the hypothalamus. The blood vessels dilate near the surface, filling with blood to allow evaporation through the normal mechanism of flushing and sweating. The blood vessels are more than usually sensitive to drops and surges in levels of estrogen and other hormones at this time.

The body notices all this flurry and checks to see why the temperature control was reset. It returns to homeostasis (balance) as soon as it can. After a while, a woman's body gets tired of playing this exciting game. It figures out how to be at peace with the lower levels of estrogen in circulation.

Osteoporosis

Osteoporosis (OP) is a big public concern. OP is the thinning of bones, often leading to pathological fractures, that is, breaking a bone without trauma, or with less than usual force in an accident. The media tell us that we're all in desperate need of calcium supplements and lots of dairy products. Are we really all about to break a hip if we're active past fifty-one years of age? While it is true that broken hips in older women are closely linked to serious breakdown of health, women are not about to break a hip when their periods get scanty. There is usually plenty of time to adjust nutrition to prevent pathological muscle and bone problems.

Only a small number of women have signs and symptoms from bone loss caused by aging. Severe osteoporosis is not linked to low estrogen levels alone. It is caused by a high-protein diet, high sodium intake, and other risk factors in combination. Seventy-five percent of postmenopausal women don't have a problem with osteoporosis, though statistics on this vary. For the twenty-five percent of women who do have problems, family history and personal health are significant in addition to menopausal changes.

Vaginal Dryness

Vaginal dryness is a concern when the spirit is willing but the flesh is, well . . . not lubricated. Dryness may be accompanied by itching of the vulva, genital burning and irritation, a thin discharge, painful intercourse, bleeding after sex, or frequency of urination or other problems signaling urinary tract irritation.

While some older medical textbooks inadvertently insult all women over age thirty-six by calling our natural changes *atrophic senile vaginitis,* menopausal women have kept their vaginas and libidos supple into their seventies. What would a thirty-six-year-old senile vagina do to deserve this outdated medical definition—keep forgetting where the car keys are? For heaven's sake!

If there is discomfort during intercourse or if vaginal dryness persists despite arousal, there may be an infection or thinning vaginal walls. Thinning walls from atrophy may be more of a problem than dryness, as this can lead to pain or bleeding with sex. Ironically, thinning is helped by sex, along with regular nutrition, including isoflavones (soy, alfalfa sprouts).

Changes in Menses

A symptom of menopause that is most changeable is the menstrual cycle itself. It can stop, start, stop again, or come in floods. Some women complain they thought they were all through, took some herbs for other reasons, and restarted their periods because of the estrogenic effects. This is particularly likely with black cohosh root or ginseng root. But no herb is strong enough to keep a woman menstruating when her eggs are used up.

Cardiovascular System Risks

The cardiovascular system (CVS) is at risk as we age, but women rely on premenopausal estrogen to prevent problems. After menopause, we must decrease our fat intake and use our physical bodies to burn off calories as well as the stress that impacts the heart. Otherwise we begin to match middle-aged men in rates of heart failure, strokes, and heart attacks. A woman's CVS risk is currently believed by conventional medicine to be in proportion to her level of estrogen. The integrated approach is that estrogen is one of many factors in calculating a woman's postmenopausal risk of heart disease.

Dysmenorrhea

Painful menstrual cycles are a symptom of menopause for some women, but it is not common for this symptom to begin only at menopause. Because there may be fibroids, polyps, ovarian cysts, or other pelvic conditions, this symptom responds to care for those conditions rather than menopausal formulas. Dysmenorrhea and pain may accompany uterine prolapse or blockage.

Depression, Stress, and Physical Pain

One of the predominant symptoms of menopause is mood change and vulnerability to stress. But despite stereotypes of frenzied middle-aged women, our stress response actually improves after an initial period of unpredictability.

In the past, ignorance and fear of women's changes caused menopausal women to be institutionalized for "involutional melancholia" as recently as the turn of the twentieth century.

Depression, aging, and arthritis all go together for some women facing menopause. Pain thresholds often change with hormonal change. Thoughts of death and suicidal feelings at any stage during menopause are not necessarily a sign of mental disease. This statement may draw fire from psychiatrists, and of course ignoring suicidal feelings is dangerous from any point of view. However, menopause is no reason to medicate or institutionalize a woman. She may be reasonably depressed, looking over her life. A "death" to what has gone before can bring on shock, grief, and recovery.

Cause

Natural (gradual) or surgical (sudden) menopause is caused by the decrease in ovarian function or by removal of ovaries, leading to lower levels of estrogen. Women's bodies have been naturally designed to have much less estrogen in later life than was required for menstruation, conception, pregnancy, and lactation. The drop in estrogen at menopause is not absolute. Even in mediocre health, there is still plenty of estrogen for continuing health.

Premature menopause is linked to smoking, illness, chemotherapy, radiation, and surgical removal of the reproductive organs. Other causes of premature menopause include malnutrition, illness involving ovarian function, and extreme stress.

Surgical Menopause

Sometimes menopause is brought on by surgery; an unprecedented number of hysterectomies have resulted in surgical menopause. The illnesses leading to those hysterectomies are pervasive on the planet.

Conventional medical belief is that leaving the ovaries in when performing a hysterectomy allows a "natural" menopause, but for many women this is not true.

Women who have their ovaries but no uterus may have symptoms of surgical menopause.

Causes of Osteoporosis

A concern about menopause causing osteoporosis (OP) in women requires a balanced view. While lower levels of estrogen are a potent cofactor of osteoporosis, it takes more than one risk factor to cause a multifactorial disease such as OP. Change what you can, so that you can relax about the few factors you may not be able to change.

Risk factors for osteoporosis include:

- family history of OP
- consuming large amounts of caffeine and soda, including diet soft drinks (more than 5 cups per day)
- drinking alcoholic beverages daily
- early menopause
- excess fat in diet, especially animal fat (meat, cheese)
- family history of diabetes
- high-protein diet
- high-sodium diet
- lack of exercise
- low estrogen
- medical history of pathological fracture (without obvious cause or usual force)
- non-black ethnic group, especially Asian and Caucasian
- not bearing children
- overweight by more than twenty-five pounds
- smoking
- steroid drugs, especially long-term use because of arthritis, asthma, auto-immune disorders
- thyroid medication (usually long-term by menopause)
- underweight by more than fifteen pounds

We all have two types of bone cells. *Osteoblasts* (literally, bone-makers) are cells that take minerals from the bloodstream and build up concentric rings of strong bone. They coexist in bone tissue with *osteoclasts*, which are constantly taking dense bone material and breaking it down to supply the bloodstream with minerals. This healthy seesaw satisfies the body's up-and-down demands for minerals, and ensures that the bones are always in the process of being replaced with "new" building materials.

Estrogen stimulates this bone-building activity at puberty, for growth spurts, through our reproductive years. We are designed to develop strong bones to pick up our growing children, or to handle the mineral loss of menses. The more bones are used, the more they thicken, as a response to body signals to prepare for more of that physical activity. Your bones will use calcium from your blood to lay down new layers of bone every time your bones feel the pull of gravity and every time you contract your muscles. No matter how much calcium you put in your mouth, your body has its own way of keeping you upright and it's been working since long before supplements for poor diet or lack of exercise were invented. Inactivity causes our bones to lose more minerals than they can pick up and make into dense bone.

Conventional Medical Care

Unless illness causes or accompanies menopause, the allopathic view is that this may not require treatment. However, it has become standard practice for women approaching or in menopause to have hormone treatment recommended.

Hormone Replacement Therapy

Some of the problems of menopause are improved by conventional treatment, but others are caused by that same approach. In the last half of the twentieth century, prescriptions of hormone replacement therapy (HRT) for most women near menopause have been linked with symptom relief and with a sharp rise in dramatic health breakdown. There are other social and medical factors for the general increase in health concerns, but HRT is a powerful weapon the medical industry has used like a new toy. HRT may help some women, but pharmaceutical firms do not have the final answer on menopause or women's health.

HRT is routinely prescribed "just in case," whether or not a woman has problems during menopause. HRT involves both estrogen and progesterone, preventing some of the cancer risk of giving estrogen alone. Estrogen replacement therapy (ERT) is not as commonly prescribed unless a woman has had a hysterectomy.

Osteoporosis

Tests for osteoporosis measure bone density in the forearm, vertebrae, or hip. It is still unclear how much bone loss in one location leads to a fracture. A CT ("cat") scan may give more information but involves a higher dose of radiation. Conventional OP treatment depends on estrogen and calcium supplementation.

Vaginal Atrophy

Treatment for vaginal atrophy includes estrogen, Premarin cream, or lubricants for sexual intercourse.

Herbal Treatment

Herbal treatment can realign our bodies with our selves. Less ideally, we can use herbal supplements as natural drugs to "fix" each symptom, whether hot flashes or irregular cycles. The "herbal drug" approach will work sometimes for some women, but the opportunity for transformation may be lost. In this section, I will provide herbal formulas, and you can purchase herbal blends "for menopause." Though these blends help, using herbal medicine more holistically (using herbs selectively, adding nutritional self-help, taking care with other risk factors) allows women to build up their health while reducing the symptoms or risk of postmenopausal problems. In this chapter, I will also teach you how to customize a formula for your own health and circumstances. This can lead to vibrant health that not only strengthens you in areas of chronic past problems, but frees your self-healing capacity to direct its energy as needed.

Herbs for Hot Flashes

Since women's blood vessels become more sensitive to sharp drops and floods of hormones during the Change, the objective of taking certain herbs is not simply reducing the symptom of hot flashes. To change hot flashes at their source, herbal therapy works both to stabilize blood vessel sensitivity to changing hormone levels, and to "even out" the overall drop in estrogen production by the ovaries.

This is accomplished mainly by supporting the adrenal function. Our adrenals provide a little estrogen as a hormonal "cushion" when ovaries produce less. Supporting adrenal function includes using adaptogens such as *Eleutherococcus senticosus* (Siberian ginseng root) and some nervines such as *Cimicifuga racemosa* (black cohosh root). This also requires herbal support for hepatic function (liver tonics) to metabolize excess circulating hormones, and attention to fat stores of estrogen in all its forms. Perhaps that is why nature made so many hormonal herbs that are also hepatics—for example, *Verbena officinalis* (vervain herb).

Palpitations (feeling your heart pound), fall roughly in the same physical arena as hot flashes and night sweats caused by hormones, heart function, and nerves. Just a few herbs with the actions of cardiovascular tonic, nervine relaxant, and hormonal tonic can reduce all three symptoms by changing the underlying cause. Examples are

Angelica sinensis (dong quai), *Leonurus cardiaca* (motherwort), *Tilia platyphylla* or *T. europea* (linden blossom), and *Achillea millefolium* (yarrow leaf, flower). These four plants have different ways to stabilize blood vessel sensitivity in response to sharp ebbs and flows in estrogen.

Because the aim is to stabilize the blood vessels' response to circulating levels of hormones, while establishing a gradual cyclical change in estrogen rather than a sharp drought-and-flood pattern, hormone balancers such as *Angelica sinensis* (dong quai root) and *Vitex agnus-castus* (chasteberry) are used, even though dong quai is said to promote estrogen while chasteberry seems to promote progesterone. Each of these has its own particular benefit, so only some of them are in the following herbal formula. If you want to use the herbs on their own, you may choose among them. No one needs them all, no matter how nice each one sounds. One herb is going to be just right.

Reducing stress is undoubtedly important to making hot flashes comfortable and tolerable. We simultaneously optimize adrenal gland health with adaptogens, which help our adrenal glands help us to adapt to current levels of stress. An example would be *Eleutherococcus senticosus* (Siberian ginseng). Others are *Borago officinalis* (borage), *Panax ginseng* (ginseng), *Glycyrrhiza glabra* (licorice), and maybe even *Urtica dioica* (nettle leaf). These five herbs and others with similar or complementary benefits improve other related areas: pain threshold and depression.

Three of the many herbal sources of phytoestrogen (a plant compound that affects our sex hormone activity) used for menopausal symptoms, including hot flashes and a dry vaginal lining, are *Trifolium pratense* (red clover blossoms), *Angelica sinensis* (dong quai root), and *Glycyrrhiza glabra* (licorice root). Licorice carries some cautions. Moderate amounts suggested in formulas in this book are conservative yet helpful for most women as an anti-inflammatory, antiviral, antibacterial, soothing herb that moistens inside and out. Because it may cause some women's bodies to retain water, licorice root is always optional; it should be omitted if there is severe water retention, high blood pressure, heart failure, or kidney failure. An excellent natural source of phytoestrogens that does not cause these problems is *Smilax spp.* (sarsaparilla root), but it is often adulterated (mixed with other herbs in commerce), so ask about purity where you buy it.

Panax ginseng (ginseng root) taken for six weeks and longer works well for symptoms of low estrogen, though it does not contain or stimulate estrogen directly. It has estrogenic effects, though it works in the short term by improving stamina and stress resistance. Over the long term it improves degenerative conditions associated with aging. Ginseng contains saponin glycosides, which have a beneficial effect on sex hormone activity. In addition, it is helpful to cardiovascular health (high cholesterol and blood pressure), nerve function, blood sugar balance, and immunity, including possible antitumor activity.

Ginseng should not be taken in cases of mental illness, or with stimulants (coffee), during hormone therapy, or during any acute stage of an illness. It does not work well for high-strung people. It is best for low-energy states. If you try ginseng and it disagrees with you, you will know because it causes headaches, palpitations, insomnia, and possibly itchy skin (*pruritus*). Discontinue ginseng use and you'll recover rapidly. It may restart periods until the body cannot naturally sustain menstrual cycles.

Some Traditional Chinese Medical Practitioners say that menopausal women should never take ginseng. I am not a traditional Chinese doctor, nor are the women who come in and tell me of the benefits it gave them. There is research that supports both views. The use of ginseng is certainly easier on a woman than HRT. The temporary "ginseng headache" is not such a terrible side effect to correct. *Panax quinquefolium* (American ginseng root) is milder and has similar effects, but it is endangered, so buy cultivated roots grown and harvested with ecological sensitivity.

The first Herbal Formula (below) is for hot flashes at nighttime. It is easier to take this tea in the middle of the night if you prepare a thermos or other container and keep it in a convenient place nearby.

Herbal Formula I

Leonurus cardiaca (motherwort herb)	½ ounce
Tilia spp. (linden flower)	1 ounce
Matricaria recutita (chamomile flower)	2 ounces
Scutellaria lateriflora (skullcap herb)	1 ounce
Salvia officinalis (sage leaf)	1 ounce
Hibiscus sabdariffa (hibiscus flowers)	1–2 ounces, to taste

Combine herbs. Use one ounce of the mixture steeped in one pint of boiling water for fifteen minutes. Strain and keep the tea in a closed container, allowing it to cool to room temperature. This tea is to be sipped while toweling off after a shower (following a night sweat) and returning to a fresh, dry bed. Drink ½–2 cups, as needed, but remember to empty your bladder before returning to sleep.

If made as a tincture, this is effective in much smaller amounts. Replace hibiscus and sage with motherwort; take ½ teaspoon every ten minutes as needed. Motherwort is an herb specific to heart palpitations as well as menopausal hot flashes and a healthy liver function. It tastes bitter, but is worth it.

Though this may seem like an undue amount of nighttime activity when fatigued, it gets you to sleep faster than lying on a damp bed while drinking ever-stronger, sleep-inducing herbs. The sleeping area should be associated with successful nights of sleeping, not nighttime wakefulness.

Hops and valerian are stronger sleep-inducing herb teas or tinctures, and they taste correspondingly stronger. Either or both may be used as tinctures; take ½ teaspoon every ten to twenty minutes as needed, for those times when the mind needs to turn off so that the body can sleep deeply. One to two cups of Herbal Formula I, taken a few hours before bedtime, prepares the body to wind down for fewer hot flashes and a less broken sleep. Remember to empty your bladder last thing before bed.

Herbs for Osteoporosis

Herbs rich in calcium and other minerals for preventing problems such as osteoporosis are best taken as a tea instead of a tincture because the water assists absorption. These teas include *Avena sativa* (oat straw herb), *Urtica spp.* (nettle leaf), *Rumex crispus* (yellow dock root), *Trifolium pratense* (red clover flower), *Medicago sativa* (alfalfa herb), *Symphytum officinale* (comfrey root and mature leaf), and *Equisetum arvense* (horsetail herb), taken as standard preparations for either leafy herbs or roots.

Herbs for Vaginal Dryness

Vaginal dryness and thinning of the vaginal lining are treated with phytoestrogen herbs, which have been described in the paragraphs on other herbal approaches for hot flashes, palpitations, and night sweats.

One problem associated with loss of vaginal lubrication is the possibility of infection. This may ascend to the bladder (cystitis), or even the kidneys. When the first warning signs of a bladder infection come on (difficulty urinating, pain on passing urine), prevent their progression with demulcents and diuretics, such as one handful of parsley chopped fresh into salads and sprinkled over cooked whole grains, daily for two weeks. Marshmallow, a soothing, cooling diuretic, may be added to antimicrobial diuretic herb teas such as yarrow or bearberry (uva-ursi); drink one to three cups a day for a minimum of three days. A repeated or severe infection that does not respond well to herbs in two to three days must be taken seriously; please see Chapter 17 on UTIs. If you cannot ask the advice of an herbalist, see a nurse-practitioner, certified nurse midwife (CNM), or other care provider qualified in women's preventive care.

Herbs for Irregular Cycles

Irregular menstrual cycles are often a woman's first sign that she is in menopause. Hormonal normalizers such as *Vitex agnus-castus* (chasteberry), *Angelica sinensis* (dong quai root), and *Cimicifuga racemosa* (black cohosh root) are the foundation for making the change graceful. Our basic approach is to promote naturally occurring levels of estrogen, look beyond symptoms that come and go, and support regular physiological function of each body system impacted by the Change.

Chasteberry is a hormonal remedy in use for women's health for over 3,000 years, dating back to Mediterranean civilizations. Herbal remedies for hormonal imbalance often contain sterols (or in the case of chasteberry, flavonoids), which are not identical to human hormones though they affect our hormone levels in ways that are not yet clear. Our mammalian biofeedback loops seem to retain control over what plant hormone is used and what is excreted. Our cells have receptor sites where our own hormones stimulate cell activity. Weaker plant hormonal compounds block the receptor site, stimulating cell activity in a far milder form.

Chinese research suggests that dong quai has two different effects on estrogen levels. It competes with estrogen for binding sites, but only when estrogen is in excess. This may allow the liver to break down the excess circulating estrogen, leading to eventual balance or decrease of estrogen. This is why dong quai is used for some women who have fibroids or reproductive problems of excess estrogen. But if there is too little estrogen in circulation, too many free binding sites go empty until the same herb compound fills those places. In this case, its presence acts enough like a weak estrogen to relieve symptoms of deficient estrogen until the body has had time to synthesize enough of its own.

Dong quai, along with *Bupleurum* and other companion herbs, was relatively unknown to Euro-American herbal traditions until the last half of the twentieth century. In Europe, older herbal practitioners with whom I interned said that they could not treat menopause so safely and effectively without the pungent seed of vitex (chasteberry). It may be that alternatives such as American ginseng, red clover, and the cohoshes were not of high quality in past decades.

False unicorn root, which is a standard American remedy, has been endangered in the wild. Only now are plant communities recovering from overharvesting, in part because ethical herbal practitioners will not use it unless they personally collect it where it is locally abundant. However, it is still named in mass-produced herb books and formulas. Nature is generous in giving us several equally good herbs in the hormone-balancing category. Chasteberry is not endangered, and is easily cultivated in warm climates.

Herbs for CVS Risk

The best herbal formula takes into account a woman's preexisting cofactors for CVS risk. The most famous herbal "foods" for the heart muscle and blood vessels are: *Crataegus spp.* (hawthorn); *Leonurus cardiaca* (motherwort) for palpitations, hot flashes, and night sweats; and *Allium sativum* (garlic) for lowering excess cholesterol, normalizing blood fats, and lessening the effects of arteriosclerosis. In addition, bitters and aromatic herbs are often cooling and beneficial to circulation. Two such herbs are *Achillea millefolium* (yarrow) and *Verbena officinalis* (vervain).

For instance, a menopausal woman with high blood pressure could use herbs noted for reducing hypertension, such as hawthorn, linden blossom, yarrow, or motherwort. But she doesn't need them all. Only motherwort is also a specific for the hot flashes and heart palpitations she may get when she is nervous. If she is not nervous but retains water, yarrow is a better tonic herb to include in her menopause formula. Improving cardiovascular health generally is what hawthorn does best, especially in preventing recurrence of strokes and heart attacks or damage to the circulatory system. Linden is mildly relaxing and soothing to the digestion, so if she has irritable bowels and menopausal symptoms along with high blood pressure, this might be her key herbal ally.

The next herb in the formula should focus on normalizing the hormonal shift rather than on a symptom (hot flash) or a constitutional area of weakness (heart and circulatory system). This brings us to the large group of hormonal tonics, including dong quai, chasteberry, and black cohosh, described earlier. These plants stimulate our body's rhythms, from a young girl's puberty to maternity, maturity, menopause, and postmenopausal rhythm.

Herbs for Dysmenorrhea

For treating dysmenorrhea herbally, we use connective tissue tonics such as *Caulophyllum thalictroides* (blue cohosh root) and *Equisetum arvense* (horsetail herb). These can help a woman heal, but it takes more than this. It's hard to have good sex when you hurt, so herbs to relax taut muscles, calm inflamed vaginal tissue, and heal thin walls are all used as part of the approach to dysmenorrhea and pain.

Many astringent and vulnerary herbs such as *Achillea millefolium* (yarrow leaf, flower) and *Calendula officinalis* (calendula flower) are digestive bitters, so they improve conditions of pelvic congestion, sluggish bowels, bloating, intestinal gas, and even heavy menstrual bleeding. Other digestive herbs with helpful bitter properties as well as hormonal support through menopausal changes are *Salvia officinalis* (sage plant), *Artemisia vulgaris* (mugwort herb), and *Verbena officinalis* (vervain herb).

Herbalists work on pelvic congestion by improving liver function rather than stimulating the colon with senna or other laxative herbs. Senna pods and other strong anthraquinone-containing laxative herbs are useful in a pinch, but they only work on a symptomatic level. They stimulate nerves in the bowel wall to empty (peristalsis), which can be harsh on the body.

Herbs for Body Pain and Depression

If body pain associated with menopause is severe, take up to one ounce of passiflora tincture, diluted in one eight-ounce cup of water or herb tea. If pain is associated with insomnia, take a cup of sleep-inducing herb tea (from mild chamomile to medium-strong motherwort to strong valerian). Only the chamomile tastes good as tea to most women, so other forms are capsules (which take up to an hour and a half to take effect) or glycerin tinctures. Some women find that one to three teaspoons of tincture, diluted in a little juice, herb tea, or water, sipped over ten minutes, does the trick in twenty minutes or less; repeated doses of alcohol tinctures for pain relief or insomnia are for short-term symptom management only.

Depression related to physical changes apparent at the time of menopause respond well to herbal therapy, especially if joint pain or arthritis is linked to feeling blue. Musculoskeletal tonics for aches and depression may be perfect since these include many herbs found in herbal formulas for menopausal women. Among the best of these are *Cimicifuga racemosa* (black cohosh), *Hypericum perforatum* (St. Johnswort), *Dioscorea villosa* (wild yam root), and even the mildly euphoric *Turnera diffusa* (damiana herb). Many of the nervines with an affinity for healthy reproductive function, such as damiana and black cohosh, are used to simultaneously relax muscles, lessen pain, and calm the nerves. This combined benefit often enables women to cope better with taxing changes related to self-image and sexuality. Long-term use of St. Johnswort is a minimum of eight weeks for its antidepressant effect. Using herbs to come off antidepressants or sedatives can be successful, though it is best done under the supervision of a qualified and sympathetic care provider who is familiar with herbs.

Creating Your Own Herbal Formula for Menopause

Most menopause formulas on the market are not the answer. The capsules or liquids seem to work well for a while, but formulas don't change in the package when your body changes. To have any effect, these over-the-counter formulas must assume a shotgun approach to hit the most common symptoms without giving women separate formulas. To avoid safety risks, most formulas designed for the average consumer have to be too mild for some women's symptoms.

Though there are seven symptoms requiring attention in the herbal treatment of menopausal women, too many herbs spoils the brew. There are three simple parts to a well-balanced herbal formula. The first is a reproductive tonic that does not necessarily alter hormones but supports a woman in broad-based ways. Gentle, general medicinal herbs for menopausal change include *Rubus idaeus* (raspberry leaf), the hormonal tonics already described, and *Anemone pulsatilla* (pasque flower herb). The reproductive tonic is the most important herb in your formula.

Secondly, what herbs will support the tonic herb with nutritive qualities? This is your helper herb. It may also help symptoms, but it provides minerals and nourishment for your heart, your liver, or all of you.

The first two herb types are rounded out with an herb directed at reducing stress and relaxing muscles, which in turn may help circulation. Nervines tone or improve nerve function, antispasmodics relax muscles, and analgesics or anodynes relieve pain. This group of herbs includes *Scutellaria spp.* (skullcap herb), *Passiflora incarnata* (passionflower herb), *Avena sativa* (oat straw herb), *Leonurus cardiaca* (motherwort herb), and *Valeriana officinalis* (valerian root).

Go down the list of seven common menopausal symptoms (see "Symptoms" earlier in this chapter) and identify the areas that concern you personally. For example, you might summarize your experience of menopause so far this way: "Hot flashes are driving me nuts. If I could just get some sleep I know I'd feel less irritable, less likely to have hot flashes all day long."

Another woman might say, "Hot flashes are no problem; I never need a sweater and it saves on my heating bill. I only get night sweats after late-night coffee or a bottle of red wine with dinner. I exercise most days, love tofu and salads, and have no risk factors for heart problems other than normal aging and menopause. But I met someone recently . . . my irregular cycle is a major problem, as I cannot take the chance of pregnancy."

A third woman says, "My nerves are shot. I hate menopause so don't even tell me what a blessing and a mysterious journey it is. I am afraid I'll get osteoporosis, and exercise makes me gag. Put nerves up near the top of the list."

The first woman may respond to herbs as simple as two daily tonics: motherwort and black cohosh (standard preparation, tea or tincture), plus two herbs at bedtime as needed: vervain and valerian (standard preparation of tinctures). Black cohosh is in many standard European and American menopause formulas because it has estrogen-like effects, decreases nervous tension, and has an affinity for decreasing joint pain and stabilizing mood swings. It also has the bonus effect of toning the respiratory system.

The woman whose cycle is irregular may only need to take chasteberry tincture each morning and drink two cups of dandelion tea every day whether she has wine for dinner or not.

The third woman wants nutritive support: nettle, skullcap, and a hormone balancer, possibly dong quai (standard preparation of tinctures) for a minimum of two months, plus education about eating soy foods, sprouts, and adequate protein at every meal. These are not prescriptions for a presumed diagnosis; this is one way to match the smallest possible number of herbs to each individual so that self-healing can take place.

In each case, herbs should bring some quick improvement of symptoms but also strengthen constitutional health. What chronic problems of constitutional health need help? Pick herbs with both an affinity for toning a weak body system and benefits specific to your menopausal symptoms.

When in doubt, start with this basic combination of herbs to cover all bases:

Herbal Formula II

Vitex agnus-castus (chasteberry seed)	1 ounce
Hypericum perforatum (St. Johnswort)	2 ounces
Leonurus cardiaca (motherwort herb)	3 ounces
Glycyrrhiza glabra (licorice root)	1 ounce

OR

Eleutherococcus senticosus (Siberian ginseng root)	1 ounce

Note: If there is any preexisting hypertension, hypokalemia (potassium deficiency), or history of renal or cardiac failure, replace licorice root with Siberian ginseng. Infuse 1 ounce of herbal mixture to 3 cups of water for twenty minutes; strain and drink three cups daily. Alternatively, combine these tinctures and take 1 teaspoon in water three times a day.

For preventing osteoporosis, add:

Angelica sinensis (dong quai root)	1 ounce
Equisetum arvense (horsetail herb)	1 ounce
Trifolium pratense (red clover flowers)	1 ounce
Avena sativa (oat straw herb)	2 ounces

For vaginal dryness or thinning, add:

Panax ginseng (ginseng root)	1 ounce

For heavy bleeding, or spotting between cycles, add:

Vitex agnus-castus (chasteberry)	1 ounce
Salvia officinalis (sage leaf)	2 ounces
Mitchella repens (partridge berry herb)	2 ounces

For preventing cardiovascular risk, add:

Crataegus oxyacantha, Crataegus spp. (hawthorn berry, leaf, flower)	3 ounces

For pain or dysmenorrhea, add:

Passiflora incarnata (passionflower herb)	2 ounces
Cimicifuga racemosa (black cohosh root)	2 ounces
Dioscorea villosa (wild yam root)	1 ounce

For depression and tension associated with painful arthritic changes, add:

Cimicifuga racemosa (black cohosh root)	2 ounces
Hypericum perforatum (St. Johnswort herb)	2 ounces
Arctium lappa (burdock root)	1 ounce

For women with surgical menopause, especially those with cancer or a history of cancer making HRT unsafe, hot flashes and mood swings can be debilitating. Here is their own combination:

Herbal Formula III

Panax ginseng (ginseng root)	2 ounces
Vitex agnus-castus (chasteberry)	2 ounces
Viburnum opulus (cramp bark)	2 ounces
Leonurus cardiaca (motherwort herb)	4 ounces

Combine these extracts and take one teaspoon three times a day, plus a dropperful (up to ¼ tespoon) for symptom relief every ten minutes or as needed.

Tea is not as practical unless one has time to prepare the different herbs properly: ginseng must be decocted for an hour, cramp bark simmered for twenty minutes, the other two herbs steeped twenty minutes (the taste is bitter).

Tea or extracts of these herbs can be used for one to three months.

External Herbal Therapies

When vaginal irritation occurs, a woman may douche if she feels she must. Use aloe gel (since aloe gel is refrigerated, you may wish to let it warm up to room temperature before use) whisked with sterile water (not just from the tap); it is very soothing for inflammation but is not drying.

An alternative is to apply yogurt for minor irritation, especially yeast. Use a teaspoon at a time, and wear a panty liner or old underwear. This may be done most easily while you lie horizontal, as when you sleep at night.

Natural lubricants can make a big difference. Wild yam oil is the basis for many natural creams used specifically in menopause for improving vaginal lubrication. But unless the herb extract is pharmaceutically manipulated in the lab, there is no evidence that wild yam has the natural systemic effect of promoting hormonal balance because of the herb's plant sterols. Wild yam used vaginally helps to relieve inflammation and dryness; it does more than lubricate, as it improves the tone or tissue integrity of the vaginal lining.

Use of lubricating aromatherapy helps us to get in touch with our bodies. Vitamin E works well, combined with sandalwood, ylang ylang, or clary sage essential (volatile) oils. To make your own, place 3 drops each of one or more of the above essential oils in ½ ounce of vitamin E, wild yam, or calendula herbal oil (see Chapter 2: Herbal Preparation). Apply a few drops to clean fingertips, and massage into labia and vaginal walls. Lubricating herb mixtures shouldn't sting or irritate; use conservatively if the skin is broken.

If vaginal use of herb oil causes redness, the essential oils may be too strong, so add more vitamin E or herb oil. Also, rinse with plain cold water and perhaps wait a few days before trying a little again. Herbs are powerful as well as gentle; a little goes a long way. These are normally so safe and beneficial that any continued irritation is a sign of something else: possible allergy, infection, or individual sensitivity. In such cases, discontinue using any preparation vaginally, and see your health care provider.

Dry or mature skin responds well to the vulnerary and moisturizing herbs:

External Herbal Formula

Symphytum officinale (comfrey root, leaf)	1 ounce
Sambucus nigra (elder flower)	1 ounce
Calendula officinalis (calendula flowers)	¼ ounce
sandalwood essential oil (optional)	10 drops

Cover ½ ounce of mixed herbs with 1 cup of boiling water; steep for ten minutes, then strain and add essential oil. Shake well, and store in a glass container in the refrigerator for up to five days. Every day, pat this herbal mixture onto damp or dry skin with a cotton pad or clean fingertips instead of using soap or cleansers. Massage lightly into the face, hairline, and neck. Rinse with clear water if desired, or leave on skin to air-dry. Repeat indefinitely as desired. Allow two to four weeks for improvements to skin tone.

Dry hair and skin can be conditioned by regular use of aromatic plants with oils and proteins.

Herbal Hair Rinse

Rosmarinus officinalis (rosemary leaf)	3 ounces
Urtica dioica (nettle seed, root, leaf)	2 ounces
Matricaria recutita (chamomile flower)	1 ounce

Cover 2 ounces of herb mixture with 1 quart of boiling water, and steep for fifteen minutes; strain and cool to a comfortable temperature. Pour 2 or more cups over hair after shampooing or each shower. Rinse with plain water or leave herbal rinse to coat ends; towel-dry hair. If tea is stored, refrigerate up to three days or add fifty drops (approximately 2 milliliters) of essential oil of rosemary or chamomile. If essential oils are used, shake well before each use; use within a few weeks or discard if it smells strange (especially in hot weather).

Gray hair can even be tinted herbally with moisturizing plants and oils. Women have been using moisturizing herb extracts such as nettles for hair care since the Ice Age, along with comfrey, rosemary, lemon grass, and chamomile. To change color, stronger plant stains have been combined with herbs in hair rinses, such as black walnut, cloves, coffee, and henna. A little goes a long way!

Henna comes in neutral, red, and other colors. Overuse of henna and water alone is drying to hair. Traditionally, 2 ounces of henna is combined with other herbs as desired, water, and plant oils (such as 2 ounces of olive or 2 tablespoons of jojoba) to make a warm mud pack; leave it on your hair for thirty to ninety minutes. Experiment and enjoy! Shampoo hair *before* rinsing with water to better remove the herbs and oil; it may take a few wash and rinse cycles. Condition with herb rinse above. Pat a few drops of essential oil of rosemary onto the tips of your hairbrush bristles and gently pull it through ends of your hair. Let your hair dry naturally. The first day after using henna, your hair may feel stiff, but from the second day on, it will shine. Repeat once every six to twelve weeks as desired, but not more than four times a year total. Overuse of henna can cause eventual allergic sensitivity, which lets you know to use the moisturizing herbs without the coloring.

Nutrition

To ease the menopausal transition, a varied, unrefined whole-food diet based on grains, fresh fruit, and vegetables in season is helpful. Especially nourishing are wheat germ, yogurt, apricots, garlic, sprouts, and old-fashioned oatmeal (not microwaved instant).

Further, women who have an easier menopause tend to avoid excess protein and phosphorous-rich foods (which increase the loss of calcium), red meat, refined flour, sugar, junk food, additives, salt, hot spices, alcohol, smoking, and caffeine (including chocolate and diet sodas).

Moderation in regard to some phosphorous-rich foods (legumes, yellow corn, nuts, parsnips) is recommended because, even though phosphorous competes with calcium, the fatty acids and phytosterols of many legumes (peas, beans) and nuts (almonds) have tremendous benefits for menopausal women.

Hot flashes can be traced to spices and other common triggers including caffeine, alcohol, dietary idiosyncrasies (whatever edible substance bothers you), and stress.

For good-quality essential fatty acids (helpful to immunity, nerves, and hormone balance), enzymes (for overall metabolism, especially good digestion of proteins), and easily digested protein, try the liberal use of home-sprouted seeds and legumes of every description. Also sold in natural food stores, these soy, sunflower, aduki, fenugreek, onion, and other live green sprouts provide an array of vitamins, minerals, phytoestrogens, and chlorophyll to sweeten the belly and the breath. Sprouted seeds, besides being rich in essential fatty acids (which nourish the skin and the immune system) and providing easily digested protein, also supply vitamin E and enzymes. Avocado, wheat germ, and flax seed are food sources of vitamin E. The cardiovascular benefit of eating these high-quality fatty acids comes from choosing these natural foods with oil in moderation.

Diuretic foods that help prevent water retention and bloating are cucumber, pineapple, parsley, watermelon, cantaloupe, and freshly grated cabbage. Vitamin B_6 found in whole grains and nuts is also a diuretic. If women have taken the birth control pill longer than three years this may decrease assimilation of B_6, so more is needed by these women, whether stressed or not.

When women have any history of hepatitis, substance abuse, or other liver damage, it is important to optimize liver function through the Change. Use milk thistle (2 teaspoons of extract or 1–2 tablespoons of seeds daily). These nutty-tasting, rice-sized brown seeds can be freshly ground in a coffee grinder and added to foods such as salad dressings and soups, or sprinkled over cooked grains.

Choose foods that are high in vitamin C (citrus fruits, rose hips jam, fresh broccoli) to help with hot flashes, and B-vitamin complex (whole grains) to ensure healthy nerves.

Nutrition for Hot Flashes

Home-sprouted seeds and nuts provide essential fatty acids, proteins, and enzymes, and are easy for menopausal women to assimilate. In a study by British researchers published in the *Lancet,* twenty-three menopausal women were given foods rich in phytoestrogens: soy flour, red clover sprouts, and flax seeds. The foods were served for two weeks and made up ten percent of the women's daily calories. After two weeks, the researchers found the degree of vaginal cell maturation (a sign of estrogen levels) had gone up forty percent. The researchers theorized that estrogen pills would be obsolete if women ate these foods regularly.

Other phytoestrogen-containing foods are pomegranates and dates, ancient food symbols of the woman as fertile goddess.

Nutrition for Osteoporosis

You are not likely to be calcium-deficient unless your diet is based mainly on meat, fatty foods, salt, and sugar, all of which encourage calcium to leave the body. We normally don't absorb most of the calcium in our food. In some vegetables (spinach, beet greens, chard), oxalic acid binds with calcium, but one cup of other dark green vegetables contains the same amount of calcium as one cup of milk or one ounce of cheese. The folk wisdom about eating spinach and similar greens in many traditional cultures is to drizzle a little lemon juice or a half-teaspoon of raw organic apple cider vinegar over them, steamed or raw. The more acidic pH makes the minerals more easily digested.

For nondairy sources of calcium, use almonds and fresh seeds (sunflower, pumpkin, and sesame, including tahini spread), dark green leafy vegetables, and especially spinach. Almonds, seeds, and vegetables such as kale, dandelion greens, watercress, and parsley are much better sources of calcium and other nutrients for mature women than milk, cheese, or standard supplements. This is partially because women need trace minerals and polyunsaturated fatty acids in plant proteins with calcium. It is also preferable to avoid the negative effects from the dairy industry's addition of bovine growth hormone (rBGH), intensive heating of the animal fats, and other processing of these products. There is also the ubiquitous use of antibiotic-laced feeds to suppress outbreaks of infection from overcrowding, not to mention the negative effects of animal fats on human physiology.

Nutrition for Vaginal Dryness or Atrophy

In a study done with forty-seven women who were taking 500 IU of vitamin E daily, two-thirds were helped; half of the group who had vaginal lesions healed. Zinc helps heal wounds, too; good dietary sources include pumpkin seeds (pepitas) and garlic.

Reproductive tonics for vaginal dryness and thinning include internal use of vitamin E, evening primrose oil, soy, and other foods or phytoestrogenic herbs (licorice root, red clover sprouts or herbal preparations) with the effect of improving tissue health.

Supplements

Some women find it useful to take 600–800 IU of vitamin E to lessen night sweats. With more than 600 IU, some people find it better absorbed if it is combined with one to three grams of vitamin C (1,000–3,000 milligrams), taken in three equal divided doses with the vitamin E. After a week, it is possible to reduce vitamin E intake to 400 IU daily. It is best not to use more than 1,200 IU daily—more is *not* better! One hundred IU daily is the conservative limit recommended if there is diabetes, hypertension, or a rheumatic heart condition.

Additionally, evening primrose oil in capsules has been found effective in European trials with women. There is also a tremendous body of anecdotal evidence in North America. "Anecdotal" pertains to a short narrative or interesting story. For example, women who say they experience evening primrose oil as helpful and safer than their HRT—that is anecdotal evidence. While most research has found the minimum dose to be in a range of eight to ten 500-milligrams capsules a day, taking less or taking the supplements sporadically seems to have little or no effect in some women. Though this is expensive, it may be effective in as little as three to six weeks, making it easier for women to afford. Some herbalists suggest that even two to four capsules a day helps some of the women with whom they've worked. Though many care providers still find eight to ten capsules a day effective in clinical practice, economizing in this way may work for some women.

Women who take calcium supplements need to balance calcium with the right ratio of magnesium and phosphorus, the way nature does in a varied, whole-food diet. Take approximately twice as much calcium as magnesium. Also balance calcium with the correct ratio of phosphorous, between 1:1 or 1:1½. This translates as 1,200 milligrams calcium, 600 milligrams magnesium, and 1,800 milligrams phosphorus. We get cramps or twinges in the muscles when the phosphorous level in the blood rises, since this always makes calcium decrease (see phosphorous-rich foods listed earlier this section). While we need both minerals, the body keeps an exact tally, so supplementing one mineral only throws off the body's balance.

Here are the suggested daily amounts, if you wish to follow them:

vitamin E: 600 IU

vitamin-B complex: B_1 50 milligrams; B_2 50 milligrams; niacin 100 milligrams; niacinamide 100 milligrams; B_5 100 milligrams; B_6 50 milligrams; B_{12} 300 micrograms; or as directed on the label

vitamin C: 1–3 grams

zinc: 15 milligrams

calcium: 1,000 milligrams

magnesium: 250–300 milligrams by itself or 500–600 with calcium (1,000–1,200 milligrams)

phosphorous: 1,000 milligrams

evening primrose oil: 8–10 500-milligram capsules for three to six weeks

Other Points

The butterfly, the spiritual symbol of the soul, represents the idea that hibernation of a kind must take place in a cocoon before life's new physical form emerges, taking flight in harmony and beauty. During menopause, women need to cocoon and renew physically or in nonphysical ways.

Menopausal women are like the mythological figure of the goddess Inanna, who matures to wield new powers only after descending on a heroic journey down into the earth to visit her "dark sister" in Hades. In psychological terms, when we face our own shadows we return to our lives with fewer hidden emotional blocks; as a consequence we may discover more of our potential, our spiritual power. This isn't always comfortable. Women need to withdraw from the regular workaday world, to be alone with their innermost thoughts. But taking time at menopause for a journey into the mysterious depths of who we are is a natural birthright. It is our rite of transformation. As we grow wiser we are important for the rest of our lives. Trading the earlier female roles for this one is not required. You can make it up as you go along, too.

Menopause may bring constitutional weaknesses to our attention, or the change may seem like total chaos and breakdown. For any body signal there are choices ranging from the simplest (rest, herbs) to the most technologically complex (HRT, surgery). Physicians, trained to look for pathology (especially as we age), are taught the complex surgical and drug options. It takes an integrated approach to women's health to explain the more conservative, nature-based methods of promoting one's own well-being.

Coming Off HRT

It is every woman's decision whether HRT is for her. There is no imperative one way or the other. Many women find HRT superfluous, even if they have not been taking care of their health scrupulously for years. Only you are responsible for your decision. Take a long look at your risk factors, weighing the advantages and disadvantages for you personally. Be realistic about the lifestyle changes you are ready to make if you want to switch to natural methods. Eating well and other aspects of health emphasized in this section are profoundly helpful, but they are a way of living, not a short-term solution.

Strictly speaking, it is not necessary to wean yourself from HRT, but it helps prevent the return of symptoms, especially hot flashes and mood changes. Many women tell me that they have become fed up and thrown the prescription away all at once. Most women are just fine when they do this, although it may be easy for one woman and hard on the next.

Take the basic Herbal Formula II, or whichever variation fits your needs, for at least four weeks along with your regular HRT cycle before starting to decrease HRT at all. During the second month, reduce the dose of HRT by one quarter. As your body adjusts to the withdrawal of external estrogen, there may be a few symptoms. Prepare for this by drinking slightly stronger or more frequent cups of herb tea or doses of extract during the second month. If there are severe symptoms, go back to the full HRT dose with the herbs for an extra month or more, until you feel ready to try again. If all is going well, reduce HRT from the three quarters dose to a half dose in the third month. Every month, drop another quarter dose. When you are only taking one quarter of your HRT along with the herbs, take the pills only every other day, then every third day. As you feel ready (your health signs stay stable as drugs are slowly reduced), go another day each week until you are taking hormones only once a week. Remember, these are powerful chemicals and the body likes rhythm. Drop your dosage at any rate, but do it with consistence and rhythm.

At any time, you may go back up to the last dose that felt comfortable through the month. At any time, you may just drop the remainder of your dose but continue with herbs for at least two more months after your last HRT dose. Especially take care with natural methods of preventing heart problems and strengthening bones.

Check your nutritional choices, ways of reducing stress, and other common sense factors. Estrogen patches cause problems with blood lipids (fats), so eat extra garlic, reduce fats in the diet (if you haven't already), and help the liver and gall bladder metabolize (with hepatic bitters such as dandelion, vervain, or motherwort) so you can handle dietary oils you still need to eat.

With hormone creams, simply use half, then none, after a month or more of taking your herbal formula and following the guidelines in the "Nutrition" section of this chapter.

Give yourself time. Look for longer periods of time without bad flashes, or better nights of sleep, or other markers you may notice. Let your physician know what you are doing, even if it is just to get confirmation that you are as fine as you feel.

Hot Flash Attitudes and Routines

The hot flash, affected by stress and other vasodilators (coffee, chili) can be transformed from an embarrassment into a pleasurable little thrill and chill. Women report that hot flashes, if they are felt at all after using herbs for a while, can be pleasurable little waves of heat. One woman describes a feeling as mild as goose bumps that she renamed "life bumps," especially at times of meaningful insight or emotion. She identifies them as a sign that she is alive and in touch with her body and her spiritual path.

Since hot flashes and sweating often feel worse at night, you may want to invest in two sets of cotton or linen bedding. Since the sheets on the bed may already be soaked by night sweats that awaken you, the strongest herbs for sleep such as valerian may not be best. It isn't recommended to use strong "knock-out" herbs to return one to sleep. You might do much better to accept a temporary break in sleep or feel groggy along with having clammy sheets.

Women report that it helps to imagine the day's problems confined to the pile of damp sheets wadded on the floor, destined for tomorrow's laundry. Have a dry change of bedding nearby to toss on the mattress. Don't bother tucking in the corners too neatly. If you feel hot, chilled, or clammy and irritable from sweating, shower with warm water, ending with cooler water. This washes sweat and salts away and changes your mood, and the cooling-off process after a shower makes you sleepy again by sending blood from peripheral vessels back to the interior.

Exercise and Osteoporosis

Exercise is far more important than calcium supplements in preventing osteoporosis. Aerobic exercise and muscle-strengthening daily activity can increase bone density and bring general health benefits to postmenopausal women (this is according to the Massachusetts Medical Society, reporting on a 1987 study in the *British Medical Journal*). It's never too late to start, but the best effects are seen in women who begin regular moderate exercise around age thirty-five and continue it throughout menopause.

Weight-bearing exercise should fit a woman's tolerance or fitness, and it should be a pleasurable discipline that can be done often. The best choices involve muscle contraction and the positive effects on your bones of gravity's pull. This includes walking, running, dancing, bicycling, and weight training. Even something as simple as good posture and a lot of walking make a big difference. Exercise and posture not only help prevent osteoporosis; they prevent some cardiovascular problems.

To be healthy through menopause it is not necessary or even recommended to focus only on weight-bearing aerobics. Other health benefits come with stretching, swimming, yoga, Tai Chi or Chi Gong (slow movements and breathing), or gardening. Also, support groups or exercising with friends makes it easier to stick to it. Become your ideal image of a strong-limbed, flexible, capable woman in her new prime.

Sexual Activity and Menopausal Symptoms

For women of all ages, sex stimulates secretion of protective mucus from vaginal walls. The blood flow to the pelvis from exercise supports the moisture balance of vaginal tissues.

Hot flashes and vaginal dryness decrease in proportion to regular sexual activity. Using energy and releasing it with healthy orgasms and a healthy attitude about our changing bodies is our best means of self-help. Libido (sex drive) does not necessarily decrease for menopausal women. For many, sex becomes a new adventure of body and soul. A woman may start a new relationship—even find the kind of sex she's always wanted. As a "treatment" for dry vaginal linings, sex is not a chore to relieve the symptom. Women's choices include solo and safe sex. Sex stimulates more than moisture; it brings germ-fighting enzymes into the vagina via mucus produced by the vaginal wall glands.

Douching

Don't douche unless absolutely necessary, as douching rinses away helpful lubrication, such as the enzyme-rich mucus that traps potential pathogens. Douching also removes healthy flora, which normally ensure that our acidic vaginal secretions prevent colonization of common opportunistic yeasts (candida). Another reason douching isn't always helpful is that repeated application of water is eventually drying, making the thinner vaginal wall of menopause (already drier) even more susceptible to infections. It is healthier to nourish vaginal tone from the inside out, as described in the "Herbal Treatment" and "Nutrition" sections of this chapter.

Appendix
HERB SUPPLIERS

The American Herb Association, The American Herbalists Guild, and The Herbal Green Pages listed in the Resources have excellent directories of several hundred sources for products, dried herbs, fresh herbs, essential oils, and more. In addition, there is a small selection of mail-order companies likely to carry some if not all of the herbs in this book.

Adaptations
P.O. Box 1070
Captain Cook, HI 96704
(808) 328-9044

Tropical medicinal herbs.

Avena Botanicals
219 Mill Street
Rockport, ME 04856
(207) 594-0694

Books, herbal products.

Blessed Herbs
Martha and Michael Volchek
109 Barre Plains
Oakham, MA 01068
(800) 489-4372

Bulk herbs.

Ryan Drum, Ph.D.
Island Herbs
P.O. Box 25
Waldron Island, WA 98297

Bulk herbs.

Earth Essentials
6849 Filbert Avenue
Orangevale, CA 95662
(916) 988-4471

Variety of essential oils.

Earth's Harvest, Inc.
Eclectic Institute, Inc.
14385 SE Lusted Road
Sandy, OR 97055
(503) 668-4120

They carry herbal vaginal suppositories.

Green Terrestrials
P.O. Box 266
Milton, NY 12547
(914) 795-5238

Books, herbal products.

HerbPharm
Box 116
Williams, OR 97544
(503) 846-7178

Herbal products, tincture formulas.

Oak Valley Herb Farm
P.O. Box 2482
Nevada City, CA 95959
(916) 268-3002

Essential oils, herb products, books.

Pacific Botanicals
4350 Fish Hatchery Road
Grant's Pass, OR 97527
(503) 479-7777

Bulk herbs.

Planetary Formulas
P.O. Box 533
Soquel, CA 95073
(800) 776-7701

Traditional Chinese, Ayurvedic, and Western herb products.

Botanical Pharmaceuticals
Silena Heron, N.D.
P.O. Box 3986
West Sedona, AZ 86340

This mail-order company is for practitioners only.

Trinity Herb Company
P.O. Box 199
Bodega, CA 94922
(707) 874-3418

Bulk herbs, herb products.

Resources
ORGANIZATIONS, EDUCATION, AND JOURNALS

Many of the organizations listed below have large databases of information regarding practitioners, suppliers of herbal products, other organizations, publications, scientific literature on medicinal herbs, conferences on herbal medicine for every interest level, and instruction in herbal medicine, including any available classes in your locale.

For plant identification, it helps to have an experienced herbalist provide initial guidance. Look in the local Yellow Pages for the Botanical or Wildflower Societies nearest to your area. There are classes and apprenticeships available in just about every herbal system from Traditional Chinese Medicine to Native American; check locally or with the organizations listed above.

American Herb Association (AHA) Quarterly Newsletter
Box 1673
Nevada City, CA 95959

The American Herbalists Guild
P. O. Box 746555
Arvada, CO 80006
(303) 423-8800

Cancer Control Society
2043 N. Berendo Street
Los Angeles, CA 90027
(213) 663-7801

The Herbal Green Pages
P.O. Box 245
Silver Spring, MD 17575
(717) 393-3295

Herb Research Foundation
1007 Pearl Street, Suite 200
Boulder, CO 80302
(303) 449-2265

The National College of Phytotherapy
Amanda McQuade Crawford, M.N.I.M.H.
120 Aliso SE
Albuquerque, NM 87108
(505) 265-0795

National Women's Health Network
514 Tenth Street NW, Suite 400
Washington, DC 20004

The Northeast Herbal Association
P. O. Box 146
Marshfield, VT 05658
(802) 456-1402

International Organizations and Centers of Learning

The Centre for Complementary Health
Director, Mr. Simon Y. Mills, M.A., F.N.I.M.H., M.C.P.P.
University of Exeter
Streatham Court, Rennes Drive
Exeter, Devon EX4 4PU
England

The National Association of Australian Herbalists
P. O. Box 65
Kingsgrove NSW 2208
Australia

The Hon. General Secretary
The National Institute of Medical Herbalists, Ltd.
56 Longbrook Street
Exeter, Devon
England EX4 6AH
(01392) 426022

The Traditional Medicines Department
World Health Organization
Geneva, Switzerland

African Herbal Traditions

The International Organisation of Traditional and
Medical Practitioners and Researchers (IOTMPR)
2205 Taraval Street
San Francisco, CA 94116

Herb Journals

American Herb Association (AHA) Quarterly Newsletter
P.O. Box 1673
Nevada City, CA 95959

Edited by Herbalist and Aromatherapist Kathi Keville.

Foster's Botanical and Herb Reviews
P.O. Box 1343
Fayetteville, AR 72702

Edited by Steven Foster.

Healthy & Natural Journal
100 Wallace Avenue, Suite 100
Sarasota, FL 34237

Edited by Michael Keenan.

The Herbal Companion
The Herb Interweave Press
201 East Fourth Street
Loveland, CO 80537

HerbalGram
P.O. Box 12006
Austin, TX 78711

Edited by Mark Blumenthal, President of the
American Botanic Council.

The Herbalist
Newsletter of the American Herbalists Guild
American Herbalists Guild
P.O. Box 746555
Arvada, CO 80006

Edited by Herbalist Robyn Klein.

The Medical Herbalism Newsletter
P.O. Box 20512
Boulder, CO 80308

Edited by Paul Bergner.

Medical Nutrition
P.O. Box 1729
Gig Harbor, WA 98335

World Research News
15300 Ventura Boulevard, Suite 405
Sherman Oaks, CA 91403

International Herbal Journals

The Australian Journal of Medical Herbalism
P.O. Box 65
Kingsgrove, NSW 2208
Australia

Herbal Thymes
P.O. Box 34
Singleton, NSW 2330
Australia

The European Journal of Herbal Medicine
5 Christchurch Road
London, N8 9QL
England

Edited by Adrian McDermott, B.S.C., M.N.I.M.H.

Planta Medica
Thieme Medical Publishers
381 Park Avenue South
New York, NY 10016

Canadian Herbal Practitioners Newsletter
302–1220 Kensington Road NW
Calgary, Alberta T2N 3P5
Canada

Bibliography

"Chaste-Tree (Vitex agnus-castus)." *Medical Herbalism* Vol. 2, 5 (September–October 1990):1.

"GLA Studies." *American Herb Association Quarterly Newsletter* Vol. IV, Issue IV (1986):12.

"Human Papillomavirus and Cervical Cancer: A Fresh Look at the Evidence." *The Lancet* (March 28, 1987): 725–6.

"Improvement in Cervical Dysplasia Associated with Folic Acid Therapy in Users of Oral Contraceptives." *American Journal of Clinical Nutrition* 35 (January 1982): 73–82.

"Oral Contraceptives and Cervical Cancer." *Journal of the American Medical Association* Vol. 259 (#18) (May 13, 1988): 2696–7.

"Plasma Vitamin C and Uterine Cervical Dysplasia." *American Journal of Obstetrics and Gynecology* 151 (1985): 976–80.

"Prevalence of Dysplasia and Cancer of the Cervix in a Nationwide, Planned Parenthood Population." *Cancer* Vol. 61 (June 1, 1988): 2359–61.

Abraham, G.E. "Nutritional Factors in the Etiology of PMS." *Journal of Reproductive Medicine* 28(7) (1983): 446–64.

Ally, M.M. "The Pharmacological action of Zingiber officinale." Proc. of the 4th Pan Indian Ocean Scientific Congress. Karachi, Pakistan, Section G, 11–12, 1960.

Amann, W. "Improvement of Acne vulgaris with Agnus castus (Agnolyt)." *Ther. d. Gegenw.* 106:124–6.

Asimov, Isaac. *The Human Body.* New York: Mentor, 1963.

Barnhart, Edward, publisher. *Physician's Desk Reference '92.* New Jersey: Medical Economics Data, 1992.

Barnes, S. and T.G. Peterson. "Biochemical targets of the isoflavone genistein in tumor cell lines." Proceedings of the Society for Experimental Biology and Medicine. 208, No. 1:103–8 (1995).

Beckham, Nancy, N.D. "Phyto-Oestrogens and Compounds That Affect Oestrogen Metabolism." *Australian Journal of Medical Herbalism.* 7, No. 1:11–16 (1995); 7, No. 2:27–33 (1995).

Bergner, Paul, ed., "Chaste-Tree (Vitex agnus-castus)." *Medical Herbalism 2,* No. 5:1,6 (1990).

Berkow, Robert, Andrew Fletcher, et al. *Merck Manual.* 15th Ed. New Jersey: Merck & Co., Inc., 1987.

Bianchi, G. et al. "Effects of gonadotrophin-releasing hormone agonist on uterine fibroids and bone density." *Maturitas,* 11 (1989): 179–185.

British Herbal Medicine Association Scientific Committee. *The British Herbal Pharmacopoeia 1996.* University of Exeter, Exeter, England: BHMA, 1996.

Brush, M.G. and M. Perry. "Pyridoxine and the Premenstrual Syndrome." *Journal of International Medical Research* 13 (1985): 174–79.

Christopher, John. *School of Natural Healing.* Provo, Utah: Biworld, 1976.

Colbin, Annemarie. *Food & Healing.* New York: Ballantine, 1986.

Consensus Statement on progestin use in postmenopausal women (Editorial). *Maturitas,* 11 (1988): 175–177.

Chow, R., J.E. Harrison, and C. Notarius. "Effects of two randomised exercise programmes on bone mass of healthy postmenopausal women." *British Medical Journal* (1987) 295:1441–4.

Culbreth, David, M.D. *Manual of Materia Medica & Pharmacology*, Eclectic Institute, Inc., Sandy, Oregon 97055, 1927.

Ellingwood, R. *American Materia Medica, Therapeutics & Pharmacognosy.* Portland: Eclectic Medical Pubs., 1983. p.347.

Evans, Dr. F.J., M.P.S., F.L.S., ed. *British Herbal Pharmacopoeia.* Bournemouth, UK.: Megaron Press, Ltd., 1983.

Felter, H.W. *The Eclectic Materia Medica, Pharmacology & Therapeutics.* Portland: Eclectic Medical Pubs., 1983. First published 1922. p.391.

Felter, H.W., and J.U. Lloyd. *King's American Dispensatory.* 2 volumes (originally published 1898). 18th edition. Sandy, OR: Eclectic Medical Publications, 1983.

Ferrannini, E. et al. "Sodium Elevates The Plasma Glucose Response." *Journal of Clinical Endocrinological Metabolism* 54:455 (1982).

Foster, Steven and James Duke. Peterson Field Guide Series: *Eastern / Central Medicinal Plants*. Boston: Houghton Mifflin, 1990.

Fuchs, Nan Kathryn, Ph.D. *The Nutrition Detective*. Los Angeles: Jeremy Tarcher, Inc., 1985.

Gaby, Alan, M.D. "Multilevel Yam Scam." *American Herb Association Quarterly Newsletter*. 12, No. 1:7 (1996).

Garland, Sarah. *The Herb Garden*, New York: Penguin, 1984.

Godwin, Sue, M.N.I.M.H., Report from the Postgraduate Seminar on Gynecology held at Regent's College, National Institute of Medical Herbalists, February 1991.

Goei, G.S. et al. "Dietary Patterns of Patients with Premenstrual Tension." *Journal of Applied Nutrition* 34 (1) (1982): 4–11.

Greenwood, Sadja, M.D. *Menopause Naturally*. San Francisco: Volcano Press, 1989.

Grieves, Maud. *Modern Herbal*. New York: Dover, 1933.

Gunn, J.D. *New Domestic Physician or Home Book of Health*. Connecticut: Moore, Wilstach, & Keys, 1861.

Hahn, G. et al. "Monchspfeffer (Monkspepper)." *Notabene Medici* 16:233–6, 297–301, April/May 1986.

Herman, C. et al. "Soybean phytoestrogen intake and cancer risk." *Journal of Nutrition* 125 (1995): 757s–770s.

Hobbs, Christopher. "Vitex: The Female Herb." *The American Herb Association Quarterly Newsletter* Vol. VII, Issue 3 (Summer–Fall, 1990).

Hoerhammer, L. et al. "Chemistry, pharmacology, and pharmaceutics of the components from Viburnum prunifolium and V. opulus." *Botanical Magazine* (Tokyo), 79, 510–525, 1966.

Holst, J. et al. "Progestogen addition during oestrogen replacement therapy—effects on vasomotor symptoms and moods." *Maturitas,* 11 (1989): 13–20.

Horrobin, D.F. "The Role of Essential Fatty Acids and Prostaglandins in the Premenstrual Syndrome." *Journal of Reproductive Medicine* 28 (7)(1983): 465–68.

Jarboe, C.H. et al. "Uterine relaxant properties of Viburnum." *Nature,* 212 (5064), 837, 1966.

Kaptchuk, Ted. *The Web That Has No Weaver.* New York: Congdon & Weed, 1983.

Kayser, H.W. and S. Istanbyulluoglu. "Treatment of PMS Without Hormones." *Hippokrates* 25:25:717.

Keville, Kathi, ed. "Cranberry Cure." *American Herb Association Quarterly Newsletter* Vol. V, Issue III, 1987, quoting *Journal of Food Science,* 51:1009–13, 1986 and *Journal of Urology,* 1986.

Keville, Kathi. *Illustrated Herb Encyclopedia.* New York: Mallard, 1991.

King, Kenneth, N.D., D.B.M., Dip. Hom. M.N.H.A.A. "Hypoglycemia and Related Clinical Conditions (Including) Pre-Menstrual Syndrome." *Australian Journal of Medical Herbalism* Vol. 2, 1 (1990): 7–8.

Kubota, S. and S. Nakashima. "The Study of Leonurus sibericus L. ii. Pharmacological Study of the Alkaloid 'leonurin' Isolated from Leonurus sibericus L." *Folia Pharmacologica Japonica*, 11 (2) (1930): 159–167.

Kuchel, D. et al. "Catecholamine Excretion in 'Idiopathic' Edema: Decreased Dopamine Excretion, a Pathological Facto." *Journal of Endocrinological Metabolism* 44:639 (1977).

Kuroda, K. and K. Takagi "Physiologically Active Substances in Capsella bursa-pastoris." *Nature* 220 (5168) (1968): 707–708.

Kuroda, K. and T. Kaku. "Pharmacological and Chemical Studies on the Alcohol Extract of Capsella bursa-pastoris." *Life Sciences* 8 (3) (1969): 151–155.

Kushi, Michio. *The Cancer Prevention Diet.* New York: St. Martins Press, pp. 160, 423–424.

Laya, M., E. Larson, S. Taplin, and E. White. "Effect of estrogen replacement therapy on the specificity and sensitivity of screening mammography." *Journal of the National Cancer Institute* (1996); 88:643–9.

Lee, John R., M.D. "Osteoporosis reversal: The role of progesterone." *International Clinical Nutrition Review* 10, No. 3 (1990): 384–391.

Lemay, A. et al. "Efficacy of intranasal or subcutaneous luteinizing hormone-releasing hormone agonist inhibition of ovarian function in the treatment of yendometriosis.z (sic)." *Am. J. Obstet-Gynecol.* 158:2, February 1988, p. 233–6.

List, P.H. and L. Hoerhammer. *Hagers Handbuch der Pharmazeutischen Praxis.* Volumes 2–5, Springer-Verlag, Berlin.

Loeb, Stanley et al. *Professional Guide to Diseases.* 3rd Ed. Springhouse, Pennsylvania: Springhouse Corp., 1989.

London, R.S., et al. *Journal of the American College of Nutrition* 3(4) (1984): 351–6.

Lutomski, J. "Chemistry and the Therapeutic Use of Licorice (Glycyrrhiza glabra L.)." *Pharmazie in Unserer Zeit* 12(2) (1983): 49–54.

Lyttleton, Jane. "Cervical Neoplasia: The Case for an Alternative to Surgery." *Journal of Chinese Medicine* No. 27.

Mabey, Richard, ed. *The New Age Herbalist*. New York: Collier, Macmillan, 1988.

Madaus, G. *Lehrbuch der Biologischen Heilmittel*. New York: Georg Olms Verlag, 1976.

Martin, et al. "Phytoestrogen interaction with estrogen receptors in human breast cancer cells." *Endocrinology* 103, No. 5(1978): 1860–7.

McIntyre, Anne, M.N.I.M.H. *Herbs For Common Ailments*. New York: Element Books, 1992.

McIntyre, Anne, M.N.I.M.H. *The Herbal For Mother And Child*. New York: Element Books.

McQuade Crawford, Amanda, M.N.I.M.H. "The Role of Phytosterols in Women's Health." Symposium Lecture, Breitenbush Herb Retreat, Oregon 1989.

McQuade Crawford, Amanda, M.N.I.M.H. "Chaparral Redeemed." Lecture, International Plant Medicine Conference, Auckland, New Zealand, 1996.

Mills, Simon, M.A., F.N.I.M.H. *The Essential Book of Herbal Medicine*. London: Arkana, Penguin Books, 1991.

Mills, Simon, M.A., F.N.I.M.H. *The Dictionary of Modern Herbalism—A Comprehensive Guide to Practical Herbal Therapy*. Rochester, Vermont: Healing Arts Press, 1988.

Moore, Michael and Daniel Gagnon. *Clinical Herbal Repertory*. Self-published, 1986.

Moore, Michael. *Medicinal Plants of the Mountain West*. Santa Fe: Museum of New Mexico Press, 1979.

Moore, Michael. *Medicinal Plants of the Desert and Canyon West*. Santa Fe: Museum of New Mexico Press, 1989.

Moore, Michael. *Medicinal Plants of the Pacific West*. Santa Fe: Red Crane Books, 1993.

Mowrey, Daniel. *The Scientific Validation of Herbal Medicine*. N.p.: Cormorant Books, 1986. (pp. 19, 206–207).

Murphy, E. et al. "Nutrient Content of Herbs & Spices." *Journal of the American Dietetic Association* 72 (1978): 174–176.

Murray, M. and J. Pizzorno. *Encyclopedia of Natural Medicine*. Rocklin, California: Prima Publishing, 1990.

Newall, C., L. Anderson, and J.D. Phillipson. *Herbal Medicines: A Guide for Health-Care Professionals*. London, England: The Pharmaceutical Press, 1996.

Nissim, Rina. *Natural Healing in Gynecology*. New York: Pandora, 1986.

Northrup, Christiane, M.D. *Women's Bodies, Women's Wisdom*. New York: Bantam Books, 1994.

Notelovitz, Morris, M.D. and Marsha Ware. *Stand Tall! Preventing Osteoporosis*. Gainesville, Florida: Triad Publishing, 1982.

Paul, Michele, R.N. *The Women's Pharmacy*. New York: Cornerstone Library, Simon & Schuster, 1983.

Pearson, C. et al. *Taking Hormones and Women's Health—Choices, Risks and Benefits*. National Women's Health Network, 514 Tenth Street, NW, Suite 400, Washington, DC 20005. 1995.

The Old Vicarage. *Foresight Pre-Conceptual Care Cookbook*, Witley, Godalming, Surrey GU8 5PN England.

Polyakov, N.G. *A Study of the Biological Activity of Infusions of Valerian and Motherwort and their Mixtures*. Moscow: Information of the first All Russian Session of Pharmacists, 319–324, 1964.

Potts, Billie. *Witches Heal*. Ann Arbor, Michigan: DuReve Publications, 1988.

Redwine, David, M.D. "The Distribution of Endometriosis in the Pelvis by Age Groups and Fertility." *Fertility and Sterility,* January 1987, Vol. 47, p.173.

Ritz, Sandra, R.N., N.P., M.P.H., M.S. "Growing Through Menopause." *Medical Self-Care* (Winter 1981): 70–4.

Romm, Aviva Jill. *Natural Healing for Babies & Children*. Freedom, California: The Crossing Press, 1996.

Romney, et al. "Retinoids and the Prevention of Cervical Dysplasia." *American Journal of Obstetrics and Gynecology* 141:890 (1981): 890–894.

Rossignol, A.M. "Caffeine-Containing Beverages and Premenstrual Syndrome in Young Women." *American Journal of Public Health* 75 (11) (1985): 1335–37.

Rothenberg, Robert, M.D. *Medical Dictionary & Health Manual*. New York: Signet, 1983.

Samuels, Michael, M.D., and Samuels, Nancy. *The Well Adult*. New York: Simon & Schuster, 1991.

Seelig, M. "Human Requirements of Magnesium: Factors That Increase Needs." *First International Symposium on Magnesium Deficiency in Human Pathology*. Paris: Springer, Verlag, 1971, p.11.

Sharaf, A. et al. "Glycyrrhetic Acid as an Active Estrogenic Substance Separated from Glycyrrhiza Glabra (liquorice)." *Egyptian Journal of Pharmaceutical Science* 16 (2) (1975): 245–251.

Shauenberg, P. and F. Paris, *Guide to Medicinal Plants*. New Canaan, Connecticut: Keats, 1977.

Sloane, Ethel. *Biology of Women*, 2nd Ed. New York: Delmar, 1985.

Smith, S. "Vitex Agnus-Castus." Trans. S. Smith. *Zeitschrift fur Phytotherapie* (July 1986).

Tierra, Lesley. *The Herbs of Life*. Freedom, California: Crossing Press, 1992.

Tierra, Michael, ed. *Essays on Herbalism; The American Herbalists Guild*. Freedom, California: The Crossing Press, 1992.

Tierra, Michael. *Planetary Herbology*. Santa Fe: Lotus Press, 1988.

Turner, Nancy J. *Food Plants of British Columbia Indians: Coastal Peoples*. Victoria, Canada: British Columbia Provincial Museum, 1975.

Uphof, J.C. *The Dictionary of Economic Plants*. Verlag von J. Cramer, 1968.

Vander, Sherman and Luciano. *Human Physiology*. New York: McGraw-Hill, 1980.

Veiga-Ferreira, M.M. et al. "Cervical Endometriosis:z Facilitated Diagnosis by Fine Needle Aspiration Cytologic Testing." *American Journal of Obstetrics-Gynecology* 157:4 (October 1987): 1, 849–56.

Vogel, Virgil. *American Indian Medicine*. Norman, Oklahoma: University of Oklahoma Press, 1970.

Warner, Phillip, M.D. "Estrogen Substitutes Aren't All the Same." *New York Times*, Letter to the Editor, Nov. 22, 1994.

Weiss, R.F. *Herbal Medicine*. Beaconsfield, England: Beaconsfield Publishers, 1988.

Whitehead, et al. "Megaloblastic Changes in the Cervical Epithelium Association with Oral Contraceptive Therapy and Reversal with Folic Acid." *Journal of the American Medical Association* Vol. 226 (#12) (1973): 1421–24.

Williams, Sue Rodwell. *Essentials of Nutrition & Diet Therapy*, 5th Ed. New York: Times Mirror/Mosby Publishing, 1990.

Wood, Matthew. *The Magical Staff*, Berkeley, CA: North Atlantic Books, 1992.

Wren, R.C. *Potter's New Cyclopedia*. 15th Ed. Saffron Walden, UK: C.W. Daniel Co., 1988.

Yaginuma, T. et al. "Effect of Traditional Herbal Medicine on Serum Testosterone Levels and its Induction of Regular Ovulation in Hyper-Androgenic and Oligomenorrhic Women." *Nippon Sanka Fujinka Gakkai Zasshi* 34 (7) (1982): 939–944.

Index

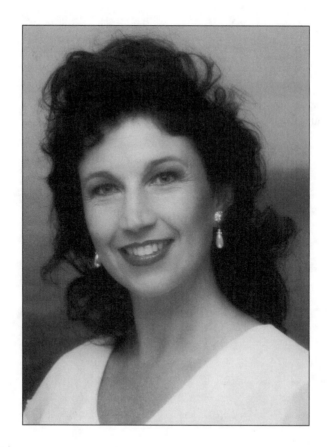

AMANDA MCQUADE CRAWFORD, member of the National Institute of Medical Herbalists, is a founding member of the American Herbalists Guild and a founder of the National College of Phytotherapy in New Mexico. She received her degree in plant medicines from England's College of Phytotherapy and has studied and taught herbal therapy throughout the world. She lives in Ojai, California.

THE HEALING POWER SERIES

With nearly 200,000 copies in print, Prima's HEALING POWER series reflects a vital new medical dialogue. Conventional physicians, practitioners of natural medicine, and the public are all coming to recognize the value of multiple approaches to health care, combining common-sense prevention and treatment with the latest tools of modern science.

The Healing Power of Aromatherapy
Hasnain Walji, Ph.D.
ISBN 0-7615-0441-9 / paperback
216 pages
U.S. $14.95 / Can. $19.95

The Healing Power of Echinacea & Goldenseal
Paul Bergner
ISBN 0-7615-0809-0 / paperback
336 pages
U.S. $15.00 / Can. $19.95

The Healing Power of Foods
Michael T. Murray, N.D.
ISBN 1-55958-317-7 / paperback
448 pages
U.S. $16.95 / Can. $22.95

The Healing Power of Garlic
Paul Bergner
ISBN 0-7615-0098-7 / paperback
304 pages
U.S. $15.95 / Can. $21.95

The Healing Power of Ginseng & The Tonic Herbs
Paul Bergner
ISBN 0-7615-0472-9 / paperback
288 pages
U.S. $14.95 / Can. $19.95

The Healing Power of Herbs, Revised & Expanded 2nd Edition
Michael T. Murray, N.D.
ISBN 1-55958-700-8 / paperback
432 pages
U.S. $15.95 / Can. $22.95

The Healing Power of Minerals, Special Nutrients, and Trace Elements
Paul Bergner
ISBN 0-7615-1021-4 / paperback
220 pages
U.S. $15.00 / Can. $19.95

The Women We Become

Myths, Folktales, and Stories About Growing Older

Ann G. Thomas, Ed.D.

U.S. $23.00
Can. $29.95
ISBN 0-7615-0654-3
hardcover / 304 pages

Through exchanges with the Old Woman who looks out at her from the mirror, Anne G. Thomas embraces the meaningful journey to old age, confronting the fears that tempt us to deny our aging. She reveals the strength and comfort that are ours if we will only acknowledge and accept ourselves as we are, and as we are becoming. Interweaving tales from the Brothers Grimm and the Bible with Native American lore and myths from Africa, Europe, and Asia, she embroiders them with insights from modern psychology to illuminate their meaning. In heartwarming style, Thomas renders a true, mythical portrait of the woman looking back at us from the mirror.

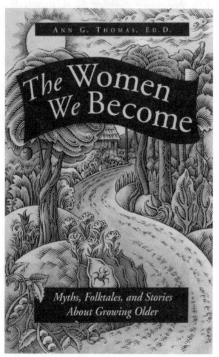

Listening to Your Hormones

From PMS to Menopause, Every Woman's Complete Guide

Gillian Ford

U.S. $18.00
Can. $24.95
ISBN: 0-7615-1002-8
paperback / 496 pages

Nearly all women will suffer from symptoms of hormonal imbalances. Some women become moody and irritable, some have panic attacks, others experience migraines, epilepsy, allergies, skin problems, low thyroid activity, ovarian cysts, or fibroids. For those with a genetic tendency toward hormonal problems, every hormonal event in life—menstruation, pregnancy, menopause—can wreak havoc. In this practical, solution-filled resource, women's health educator Gillian Ford empowers women with the facts. *Listening to Your Hormones* illustrates the pervasive role hormones play in women's lives and reveals how to form a successful partnership with a doctor to find treatments that work.

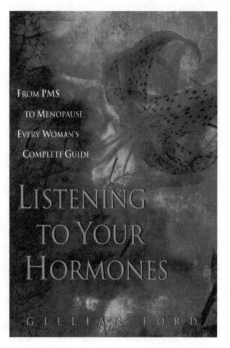

To Order Books

Please send me the following items:

Quantity	Title	Unit Price	Total
_____	_____	$ _____	$ _____
_____	_____	$ _____	$ _____
_____	_____	$ _____	$ _____
_____	_____	$ _____	$ _____
_____	_____	$ _____	$ _____

Shipping and Handling depend on Subtotal.

Subtotal	Shipping/Handling
$0.00–$14.99	$3.00
$15.00–$29.99	$4.00
$30.00–$49.99	$6.00
$50.00–$99.99	$10.00
$100.00–$199.99	$13.50
$200.00+	Call for Quote

Foreign and all Priority Request orders:
Call Order Entry department
for price quote at 916/632-4400

This chart represents the total retail price of books only (before applicable discounts are taken).

Subtotal $ _____

Deduct 10% when ordering 3-5 books $ _____

7.25% Sales Tax (CA only) $ _____

8.25% Sales Tax (TN only) $ _____

5.0% Sales Tax (MD and IN only) $ _____

Shipping and Handling* $ _____

Total Order $ _____

By Telephone: With MC or Visa, call 800-632-8676 or 916-632-4400.
Mon–Fri, 8:30-4:30.

WWW: http://www.primapublishing.com

By Internet E-mail: sales@primapub.com

By Mail: Just fill out the information below and send with your remittance to:

**Prima Publishing
P.O. Box 1260BK
Rocklin, CA 95677**

My name is _____

I live at _____

City _____ State _____ ZIP_____

MC/Visa#_____ Exp. _____

Check/money order enclosed for $_____ Payable to Prima Publishing

Daytime telephone _____

Signature _____